Acta Neurochirurgica
Supplements

Editor: H.-J. Reulen
Assistant Editor: H.-J. Steiger

Acta Neurochirurgica
Supplements

Editor: H.-J. Reulen
Assistant Editor: H.-J. Steiger

Functional Rehabilitation
in Neurosurgery and
Neurotraumatology

Edited by
K. R. H. von Wild
In collaboration with M. Lipovšek,
A. D. Mendelow, and J.-L, Truelle

Acta Neurochirurgica
Supplement 79

SpringerWienNewYork

BS

Univ-Prof. Dr. Klaus R. H. von Wild
Clemens Hospital, München, Germany

© 2002 Springer-Verlag/Wien

Printed in Austria

Typesetting: Asco Typesetters, Hong Kong
Printing: A. Holzhausen, A-1140 Wien
Binding: Fa. Papyrus, A-1100 Wien
Printed on acid-free and chlorine-free bleached paper
SPIN: 10854192

With 33 partly coloured Figures

CIP-data applied for

ISSN 0065-1419
ISBN 3-211-83739-6 Springer-Verlag Wien New York

4/19/03

Preface

Rehabilitation in Neurosurgery is not a new task but rather an indispensable part of neurological surgery from the beginning, intended to avoid or to improve diagnosable or impending damage to the CNS, and to prevent secondary and tertiary complications by adequate therapeutic measures. Rehabilitation should start right at the onset and site of the acute impact to the brain, spinal cord or peripheral nerves. Thanks to the tremendous progress in modern neurosurgery regarding microsurgical techniques, instruments, sophisticated technologies, multidisciplinary team approaches, neuro-imaging, neuropharmacology, antibiotics, neuroanaesthesiology, and intensive care treatment, more and more patients frequently survive even life threatening lesions to the brain and spinal cord, however, at the expense of severe sensory, motor and neuropsychological deficits, and long lasting disabilities. Therefore neurosurgeons taking care of the acute treatment, e.g. sophisticated operations in tumour and vascular pathology or neurotraumatology, have to be aware of the early and late sequelae. This means that neurosurgeons should be made familiar with neurorehabilitative measures to protect patients from secondary and tertiary complications and to facilitate the natural progress of recovery by restoration and compensation.

Functional electrical stimulation, neuromodulation, bio-implants and neuroprosthesis open up a most important field of functional neurosurgical rehabilitation covering movement disorders, spasticity, epilepsy, pain, and vegetative state. During the past years neurosurgeons have become increasingly involved in the broad *spectrum of neurorehabilitation* and have established special units associated with their neurosurgical institutions. As a typical example a unit for Neurosurgical Rehabilitation was set up in my department and a special clinic, respectively, near Münster, Germany. Therefore the delegates of the WFNS Committee on Neurorehabiliation, established in 1997, decided to organise the first International Conference on Neurosurgical Rehabilitation in Münster, offering the opportunity to visit various types of neurosurgical rehabilitation facilities. During this conference it became apparent that neurorehabilitation had been neglected by most of the neurosurgeons around the world during the second half of the last century and it was agreed to improve on this situation by publishing the results of their work as a special volume.

Selected papers from another two meetings (the 5th Annual Meeting of the Euroacademy of Multidisciplinary Neurotraumatology, organised in conjunction with the Meeting of the European Brain Injury Society and France Traumatism Cranien, Paris, organized by the Congress President Jean Luc Truelle, on September 20–23, 2000; Workshop on Early Rehabilitation, Maribor, Chair Matej Lipovšek, March 29–31, 2001) were collected to present a comprehensive overview of concepts, strategies, state-of-the-art treatment and results of early and longlasting neurorehabilitation and reintegration into the social environment. The authors are neurosurgeons, neurologists, neuropsychologists and members of neighbouring disciplines, all deeply engaged in modern neurorehabilitation work.

If this issue contributes to propagate modern and future orientated findings in the field of rehabilitation in neurosurgery and neurotraumatology, and, by its multidisciplinary approach, helps to improve the quality of life of patients suffering from TBI and SCI impairments, it will have fulfilled its purpose.

This first volume in a new series on Rehabilitation in Neurosurgery will be a first step in that direction, and we all are very grateful to H. J. Reulen, Editor of the Supplement Volumes of Acta Neurochirurgica, and Springer Verlag Wien to publish this special issue on Rehabilitation in the Proceedings Series of Acta Neurochirurgica, the European Journal of Neurosurgery. We extend our thanks to all authors who did their best to make this supplement a success, especially J. L. Truelle and D. Mendelow as well as M. Lipovšek, my co-workers, for reviewing the papers. In particular thanks to the personal commitment and circumspect management of Mrs. I. Anders, and Mrs. S. Schilgerius from Springer Verlag Wien and last but not least, Mrs. G. Kühling, my secretary, to eventually make this volume a success.

Financing of an international congress and the subsequent proceedings has always been a great problem, particularly so in neurorehabilitation. We therefore express our gratitude especially to Dipl. Ing. Dr. h.c. Ferdinand Piech, President of the Volkswagen AG, for his commitment as well as Dr. Christian Ebenezer, IPSEN-Pharma for his personal involvement and generous support.

Klaus R. H. von Wild
Chairman of the WFNS Neurorehabilitation
Committee
President of the EMN
Incoming Chair of the EFNS-Scientists Panel on
Neurotraumatology

Contents

Listed in Current Contents

Part I: Neurosurgical Rehabilitation, Current Concepts, Strategies, and Outcome

Acta Neurochir (2001) [Suppl] 79: 3–10
© Springer-Verlag 2001

Neuro-Rehabilitation – a Challenge for Neurosurgeons in the Century 21st Concepts and Visions of the WFNS-Committee on Neurosurgical Rehabilitation

Klaus R. H. von Wild

Clemenshospital, Teaching Hospital of the Westphalian-William's University, Münster, NRW, Germany

Summary

Objectives. Patients with severe brain, spinal cord and peripheral nerve lesions today survive surgery. This, however, is quite often achieved at the burden of disabilities. Neuro-rehabilitation could improve significantly patient's quality of life (QoL).

Methods. Formed in 1997, the WFNS Committee supports all efforts regarding personal and regional activities, teaching, research, recommandations, guidelines, and practical application to improve neurosurgeon's quality management within the spectrum of rehabilitation around the world.

Results. Neuro-rehabilitation became part of the scientific programmes at the 11th EANS, 10th AANS, ICRAN 1999, and now 12th WFNS congresses. The first international conference on Neurosurgical Rehabilitation took place in D – Münster, 2000.

Conclusions. The WFNS Committee can influence neurosurgeons to take over the challenge of neuro-rehabilitation to improve patient's outcome in respect to ICIDH-2 WHO classification. Delegates of all neurosurgical societies are kindly invited to join us.

Keywords: WFNS-Committee; neurorehabilitation; modern neurosurgery; TBI and SCI; Quality of Life (QoL).

Introduction

The obligation of a state to reintegrate the sick and injured into vocational life and the commitment to give these people support was first defined in the French constitution in the wake of the enlightenment of the French Revolution and the accompanying upheavals of the social conditions, resulting in the emergence of early models of social medicine in the modern-day sense of the term [5]. The wish and requirement for rehabilitation (Latin: "habilis" and "habilitare") in the context of "apt" and "appropriate" is, in terms of the new five dimensional ICIDH-2 Classification regarding impairment, disability, handicap, and social relationship, just as old as the endeavours to heal diseases and injuries and the wish to continue living and working in one's own social environment which were reported even as long as 5000 years ago. History teaches us that progress and renewal emerge in a society always only as a response, in other words as a direct reaction to specific demands of a certain limited time span, and in dependence on regional, continental, and – in these days of globalisation – now also world wide requirements or challenges. An exemplary case in this regard is the history of modern neurological rehabilitation in connection with neurotraumatology over the past 100 years, as an immediate reaction first to the events of the First and Second World Wars for the acute care and rehabilitation of both military and civilian victims, while today – in the wake of ever-increasing industrialisation and prosperity – it is the victims of road traffic, personal violence, spare time sports – related accidents or in accidents occurring at work or at home as a consequence of special social circumstances, possibilities, and requirements. Today more and more patients with severe brain, spinal cord, peripheral nerve lesions with or without multiorgan lesions (mainly after accidents but also after severe surgical operations) survive, however quite frequently with severe handicaps. This is achieved thanks to the development of modern surgical strategies and improved methods of surgery, neuroradiology and neurointensive care medicine [3, 6, 13–15].

Above all it is the neuropsychological disability and handicap that severely affects patients' Quality of Life (QoL) [2, 12]. Therefore these great strides which are made by modern technology and experimental basic research demand that neurosurgeons occupy themselves with functional neurorehabilitation more intensively as was postulated already by the well known neurologist and neurosurgeon Otfrid Foerster (1873–1941) [4]. During the second half of the last century neurosurgery was focused mainly on surgical and technical aspects while nowadays our interest should also be concentrated on basic research and experimental neurosurgery regarding neuroplasticity, regeneration, reorganisation, and repair [9], including biotechnology and – engineering, reconstructive techniques and functional electric stimulation in movement disorders, pain, and in comatous and VS patients [8]. Therefore neurosurgical rehabilitation became a challenging task and part of an interdisciplinary approach in this field [2, 7, 10, 11, 12]. The purpose of this presentation is to underline the important role of neurosurgery in neurorehabilitation in the future and to announce the WFNS Committee to all neurosurgeons around the world, and at the same time to invite research groups and institutions working in the field of neurorehabilitation to interdisciplinary and even transdisciplinary co-operation and scientific exchange.

Material and Methods

The objective of comprehensive neurosurgical rehabilitation is to avoid or minimize secondary damage and also tertiary sequelae whilst preserving and utilizing the available or residual neural plasticity and the individual rehabilitation potential resulting from this. This is the basis for the development and promotion of suitable replacement strategies in simultaneous suppression of repair processes impairing function. These processes can be detected and followed today by biochemical (microdialysis), electroneurophysiological (neuromonitoring) methods and functional imaging diagnostics (MRI, PET-Scans) in humans and analogous in comparative animal experiments. The Committee for Neurosurgical Rehabilitation would like to coordinate the existing approaches to research and results obtained so far in order to promote and intensify the exchanges of scientific ideas on the one hand and on the other hand to take into account the requirement for quality assurance by working out guidelines in this important field of neurosurgery all over the world. Thus modern rehabilitation medicine looks for answers to partly long-standing questions such as the actual rehabilitation potential and its utilization by external sensorimotor stimulation and coordination of multimodal operation as well as answers to compelling topical questions e.g. the significance of genetic predisposition and sex-specific behaviour as a prerequisite for repair, regeneration and functionally appropriate survival of damaged tissue as well as with regard to the patients themselves, above all how to influence their impairment most favourably to avoid a handicap and thus to improve the expected quality of life by reintegration into family, society and occupation. This of course differs widely from one continent to the other but also from one country to the other due to varying socio-economic and cultural factors.

The ad-hoc Committee on Neurorehabilitation was instituted by the WFNS on occasion of its World Congress in Amsterdam in 1997 [16]. All WFNS Member Societies were invited to nominate one delegate to participate in this challenging project. 42 delegates have been appointed up to now (Table 1). Thanks to Prof. Flemming Gjerris, President of the 11th EANS-Congress in Copenhagen, we had our constitutional meeting at the Neurosurgical Clinic of the University in Copenhagen during the 11th EANS-Congress on Sep-

tember 21st, 1999. At this meeting Matej Lipovsek, the Head of the Neurosurgical Department at the Hospital of the University in Maribor, Slovenia, accepted to act as a secretary being mainly responsible for the western half of the neurosurgical globe, whereas for the eastern half Wai S. Poon, Prof. and Chief Division of Neurosurgery, Prince of Wales Hospital, Shatin, New Territories, Hong Kong was elected at the 2nd meeting of the 10th AANS Congress in Lahore November 9th, 1999. Prof. Flemming Gjerris as well as Prof. Iftikhar Ali Raja were so kind as to follow the wish of the Committee to organise a special scientific session on neurosurgical rehabilitation as part of their official programme with Excellent lectures by invited speakers from Europe and from Asia. To co-operate with the WFNS Committee on Neurotraumatology, Congress President Mr. Wen Ta Chiu, Prof. and Superintendent Taipei Medical College, included one main session in the ICRAN (1999) scientific programme on neurosurgical rehabilitation as well the 3rd meeting of the delegates, when Prof. Yoichi Katayama, Head Department of Neurological Surgery, Nihon University Hospital, Tokyo, Japan was elected representative for functional rehabilitation in neurosurgery on November 23rd, 1999.

Results

Neurosurgical rehabilitation has become a challenging task for the 21st century. Up to now 42 delegate have been nominated. (Table 1).

From July 30th to August 2nd, 2000, the first conference on neurosurgical rehabilitation took place in Münster at the University Castle, Germany. It was organised as a WFNS Neurorehabilitation Committee Satellite Symposium on the occasion of the World Exhibition EXPO 2000 in Hanover and its World Congress on Medicine and Health, Medicine Meets Millennium (Fig. 1). Main topics were:

1) Neurosurgical rehabilitation, current concepts, strategies and outcome (21 lectures); 2) functional neurosurgery and neuromodulation (16 lectures); 3) Botulinum toxine A in neurosurgical rehabilitation (9 lectures); 4) the guided poster session "Meet the Experts"; 5) one and a half day excursion and visit of 3 different sites for modern neurosurgical rehabilitation with hands on workshops:

a) Department of Neurological Clinic for Neurorehabilitation Hessisch Oldendorf, Head Wolfgang Gobiet, M.D., Neurosurgeon, Neurologist; 345 patients: 150 beds for early (postacute) rehabilitation classified as Phase B and C, 195 beds Phase D for long time rehabilitation and Phase E respectively, concerning vocational rehabilitation in respect of the re-employment of the patients later, which is classified according to VdR, the German Social Pension and Insurance Companies,

b) Clinic Hattingen-Holthausen for Neurosurgical Rehabilitation, Head Werner Ischebeck, M.D.

Table 1. *Members of WFNS Neurorehabilitation Committee, (March, 2001)*

Ahmed Fawed Pirzad	(Kabul, Afghanistan) Afghan. Neurosurg. Soc.
Eduardo A. Karol	(Buenos Aires, Argentina) Sociedad de Cirurgia Neurologica del Cono Sur
Günther Lanner	(Klagenfurt, Austria) Austrian Neurosurg. Soc.
Marcos Massini	(Lago Norte, Brazilia) Braz. Soc. of Neurosurg.
Wolfgang Mauersberger	(Santiago de Chile, Chile) Sociedad de Neurochirurgia de Chile
Chung-Jiang Yu	(Beijing, PR China) Chinese Neurosurg. Soc.
Ninoslav Pirker	(Zagreb, Croatia) Croatian Neurosurg. Soc.
Jaroslav Plas	(Prague, Czech-Republika) Czech Neurosurg. Soc.
Ole Osgaard	(Copenhagen, Denmark) Denish Neurosurg. Soc.
Carsten Kock-Jensen	(Aalborg, Denmark) Scandinavian Neurosurg. Soc.
Adel Eisa	(Alexandria, Egypt) Egypt Soc. of Neurosurg.
Philippe Decq	(Crètail, France) French Soc. of Neurosurg.
Wolfgang Gobiet	(Hessisch Oldendorf, Germany) German Soc. of Neurosurg.
Klaus R. H. von Wild	(Münster, Germany) German Soc. of Neurosurgery
George Foroglou	(Thessaloniki, Macedonia Hellas) Hellinic Neurosurgical Soc.
Wai S. Poon	(Shatin, Hong Kong) Hong Kong Neurosurg. Soc.
K. V. R. Shastri	(Bangalore, India) Neurolog. Soc. of India
Yoichi Katayama	(Tokyo, Japan) JCNS
Takeshi Kawase	(Tokyo, Japan) Japan Neurosurg. Soc.
Nasri J. S. Khory	(Amman, Jordania) Jordan Neurosciences Soc.
Janis Ozolinsh	(Riga, Latvian) Latvian Association of Neurosurg.
Rimantas Vilcinis	(Kaunas, Lithania) Lith. Neurosurg. Soc.
Mirko Mircevski	(Skopje, Macedonia) Macedonien Neurosurg. Soc.
A. El Khamlichi	(Rabat, Marokko) Maroccan Soc. of Neurosurg.
Hans Van der AA	(Enschede, Netherlands) The Netherlands Soc. of Neurosurgeons
M. Tayo Shokunbi	(Ibadan, Nigeria) Nigerian Soc. of Neurosciences
Ingunn R. Rise	(Oslo, Norway) Norwegian neurosurg. Soc.
Iftikhar Ali Raja	(Lahore, Pakistan) Asian-Australasian Soc. of. Neurolog. Surgeons
Jan Haftek	(Warszary, Polen) Polish Soc. of Neurosurg.
Carlos Ferro	(Lisboa Portugal) Portugese Neurosurg. Soc.
Alexander V. Ciurea	(Bucharest, Romania) Romanian Soc. of Neurosurg.
Mohamed Al Joharji	(Riyadh, Kingdom of Saudi Arabia) Middle East Neurosurg. Soc.
Ahmad Ammar	(Al-Khobar, Kingdom of Saudi Arabia) PANS
Matej Lipovsek	(Maribor, Slovenia) Slovenian Neurosurg. Soc.
Freddie Kieck	(South Africa) South Africa Neurosurg. Soc.
R. Heilbronner	(St. Gallen, Switzerland) Swiss Soc. of Neurosurgery
Alexander Dah-Jium Wang	(Taipei, Taiwan) Taiwan Neurosurg. Soc.
Hakan Caner	(Ankara, Turkey) Turkish Neurosurgical Soc.
Mehmet Hacihanefioglu	(Istanbul, Turkey) Turkish Neurosurgical Soc.
Vitaly J. Tsumbaliuk	(Kiew, Ukraine) Ukrainian Assoc. of Neurosurg.
Bakulesh Soni	(Southport, UK) Neurosurgical Soc. of UK
Michael Carey	(New Orleans USA) American Assoc. of Neurological Surgeons (AANS)
Stehan Haines	(Charleston, USA) The Society of Neurological Surgery
Nguyen Van Toan	(Hanoi, Vietnam) Neurosurg. Soc. of Vietnam
Kazadi K. H. Kalangu	(Harare, Zimbabwe) Pan African Association of Neurological Sciences

Prof. and Chair Neurosurgical Rehabilitation, Private University of Witten-Herdecke, 60 beds for children, 210 beds for adults (Phase B and C), and

c) Department for Posttraumatic Early Rehabilitation at the Neurosurgical Clinic, Clemenshospital, Münster (Fig. 2): 20 beds for adults Phase B, which was a pilot project of the Ministry of Labour, Social Affairs and Health, NRW, Germany. The design of this first department for early rehabilitation as part of a neurosurgical clinic followed the Guidelines of the German Task Force on Neuro-logical/Neurosurgical Rehabilitation, as published in 1993. All rooms for patients, relatives, and staff members of the multidisciplinary team, belonging to this department only, and all diagnostic and therapeutic facilities are on the same 1st floor and next to the x-ray department with the ICU-ward above on the second floor.

17 delegates and representatives took part in the official annual meeting of the Committee (Fig. 3) to exchange their experiences with different socio-cultural

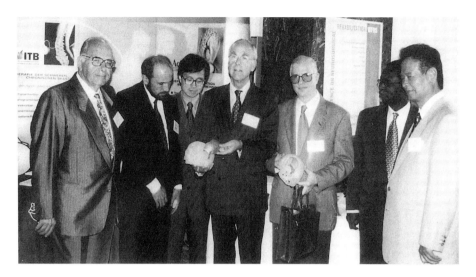

Fig. 1. Delegates visiting the industrial exhibition during the first international conference of the Committee, Münster Castle, August 1st, 2000. K. von Wild demonstrates a specially tailored titanium implant which was manufactured computerassisted preoperatively to reconstruct a large skull bone defect secondary to decompressive craniotomy because of posttraumatic malignant intracranial hypertension. From left to right. George Foroglou, Ahmed Pirzad, Wai S. Poon, Klaus von Wild, Iftikhar Ali Raja, M. Tayo Shokunbi, Tetsuo Kanno

possibilities and treatment modalities and to discuss the state of the art to formulate the future aims in neurorehabilitation. The Committee's recommendations were as follows:

1. Scientific activities: 1.1. make use of local/regional/international congresses (e.g. WFNS Sydney 2001) and executive meetings like ICRAN (bi-annual, next one will be in Bali, Indonesia, 2002). 1.2. Funding and politics: Symposium and Workshop as part of an international neurosurgical congress or satellite meeting do not require a lot of funding, and commercial sponsors are usually willing to support them. Sponsorships for travelling expenses of delegates from developing countries who will help to carry indication and know-how to where it is needed most will be the subject of this Committee: a few at a time depending on the generosity of our sponsors. 1.3. Scientific contents of the neurorehabilitation symposia and workshops should include: conventional neurorehabilitation and functional neurosurgical procedures focussing on indications and clinical outcome. 1.4. Target ordinance are young neurosurgeons.

2. Clinical applications: 2.1. Conceptually, as early as possible. 2.2. Requires a multidisciplinary team. 2.3. With a leader who could be a neurosurgeon. 2.4. To promote neurorehabilitation to young neurosurgeons as carriers of development as their special interest. 2.5. To develop, document, and define a set of common vocabulary for clinical practice and communication

in neurorehabilitation. The consensus statements will be published on the neurorehabilitation page of the WFNS web site.

3. Basic research: 3.1. Clinical outcome, measures and assessment of Quality of Life. 3.2. Modern technology, bio-engineering, neuroprosthesis, gentechnology regarding regeneration and repair of the central and peripheral nervous system, functional electric stimulation in central movement disorders, para- and tetraplegia with neuroimplants and programmes for mental, cognitive and behavioural stimulation and training make neurosurgical neuro-rehabilitation a challenge for young neurosurgeons in the future. The reality of different socio-economic, cultural and health care systems has its impact on the introduction and realisation even of simple basic concepts in neurorehabilitation, so that we all have to discuss these facts to support the delegates by inviting them for special training and education. We are looking forward to realising this challenge in neurorehabilitation in neurosurgery with great enthusiasm. We therefore invite all delegates and people to be nominated by their societies in due time at the 12th World Congress in Sydney, where, thanks to the Congress President, Prof. Dr. Noel G. Dan, and his Programme Director, Prof. Dr. Andrew Kaye, we will be able to organise for the first time a main session on neurosurgical rehabilitation. This will be a great step forward in the development of modern neurosurgery. All delegates are invited to meet there.

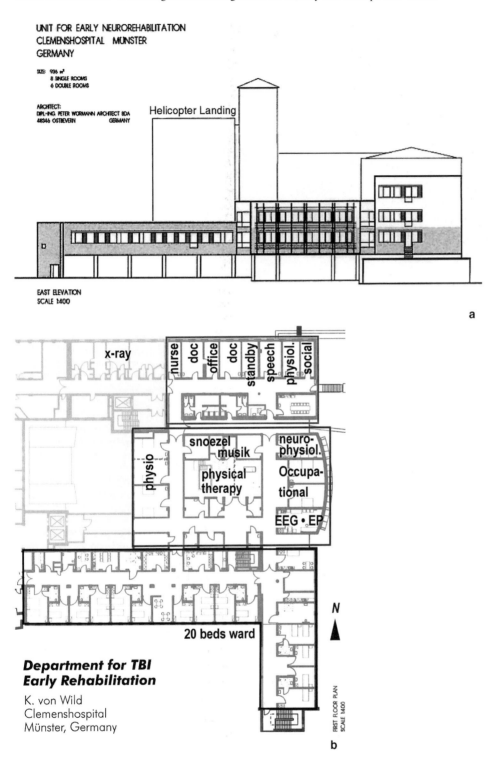

UNIT FOR EARLY NEUROREHABILITATION
CLEMENSHOSPITAL MÜNSTER
GERMANY

SIZE: 936 m²
8 SINGLE ROOMS
6 DOUBLE ROOMS

ARCHITECT:
DIPL.-ING. PETER WÖRMANN ARCHITECT BDA
48346 OSTBEVERN   GERMANY

Helicopter Landing

EAST ELEVATION
SCALE 1:400

a

x-ray

nurse · doc · office · doc · standby · speech · physiol. · social

snoezel · musik · neuro-physiol.

physio · physical therapy · Occupa-tional

EEG · EP

20 beds ward

N

**Department for TBI
Early Rehabilitation**

K. von Wild
Clemenshospital
Münster, Germany

FIRST FLOOR PLAN
SCALE 1:400

b

Fig. 2. Department for Early Neurorehabilitation, Neurosurgical Clinic Clemenshospital (Architect Dipl. Ing. Peter Wörmann BDA, D-48346 Ostbevern). Upper part shows the ground-plan of approx. 1000 m² of the novel department on the first floor with all rooms, which are connected by short access. Offices to the north, next to the x-ray department, and bed-rooms to the south-east, L-shaped. All necessary therapeutic and diagnostic facilities in the middle, next to the 2 elevators and 2 staircases

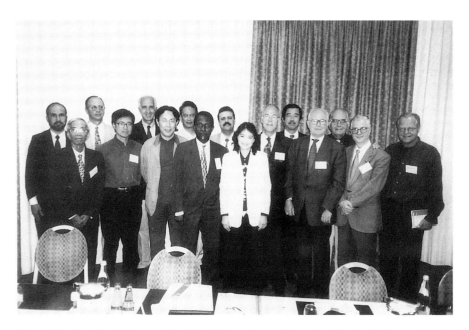

Fig. 3. Meeting of the Delegates of the WFNS Committee on Neurorehabilitation, Münster, July 30th, 2000, from left to right: Ahmed Fawad Pirzad, Nguyen Van Toan, Rimantas Vilcinis, Wai S. Poon (coordinator for Asia), Matej Lipovsek (Secretary), Alexander Dah Jium Wang, Tetsuo Kanno, M. Tayo Shokunbi, Mohammed Al Joharji, Joko Kato, Klaus R. H. von Wild, Takeshi Kawase, Hans Erich Diemath, George Foroglou, Iftikhar Ali Raja, Hans van der Aa

Discussion

The technological advances in microsurgery and intensive care and the progress made in the fields of microelectronics, computer technology, and telecommunications as well as the availability of new, constantly improved materials-to name just a few of the most important pillars – have not less than revolutionized the diagnosis and therapy in neurosurgery over the second half of the last century. The neurosurgical societies have reacted accordingly by founding special working committees, e.g. on neurotraumatology, just as our novel WFNS ad-hoc-Committee on neuro-rehabilitation as a measure to support the activities to meet with the challenges of our times by critically analyzing and discussing the goals that have already been achieved and the foreseeable progress by promoting cooperation and coordination [3, 6].

When looked at from this viewpoint it seems logical – indeed, even imperative – for us neurosurgeons to intensively devote our attention to aspects of neuro-rehabilitation now that as a consequence of the progress made more and more patients survive their highly dangerous diseases thanks to the art of modern medical management and progress in rescue, first aid, intensive care as well as in diagnostic facilities including functional MRI and PET-Scan. In many cases, how-

ever, these people survive at the price of considerable functional impairments of individual organs and organ systems, disabilities or handicaps with restrictions in their daily life and society, dependent on the sex of the person, his/her age, and social cultural factors. The reintegration of disabled persons in the family, society, and professional life constitutes the ultimate aim of our postulated and already practised holistic rehabilitation concept, one that has been acknowledged as being correct and indispensable, one that covers the entire *spectrum of neurorehabilitation* (Fig. 4) [12] starting from the rescue of the patient at the site of the accident, respectively the impact on the brain and spinal cord, acute haemorrhages or infections and his/her acute life-saving treatment (figure 4). Here we are fully aware that the mentioned requirements of the patient and above all the economic and social conditions prevalent in his/her country as well as in the regions of our modern world have their own specific laws, laws we are obliged to observe, but which we should also do our best to improve at the same time.

Assessment of rehabilitation strategies and treatment methods presupposes a close multiprofessional cooperation with all the occupational groups participating in the process of rehabilitation, i.e. the neurosurgeon to cooperate with his co-responsible specialist colleague and with nonmedical therapists, behav-

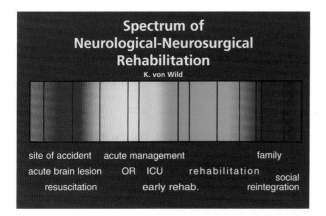

Fig. 4. Spectrum of neurological-neurosurgical rehabilitation. Starting at the site of the impact all rehabilitative measures necessary are offered to the patients according to his/her individual situation of recovery which can be characterised like the physical Frauenhofer lines of the sun-light spectrum. This spectrum differs from one patient to another as does the severity of the lesion and restorative potential

ioural neurologists, psychologists, bioengineers, neuropathologists and basic researchers from experimental sectors. In our view, neurological-neurosurgical rehabilitation already begins immediately after the occurrence of the lesion, i. e. diagnosis of sustained motor, sensory and neuropsychological damage. In the meantime, guidelines for concepts of early rehabilitation have been developed while guidelines and reviews on TBI management do not recommend the necessity of early or neurorehabilitation in case of impaired CNS functions. We do not only see the imperative need for qualified postgraduate training of younger colleagues, but above all we should be prepared to assume own responsibility for this ever more important field of neurosurgical therapy: acute, early and long-term rehabilitation. Examples are computer-assisted planning and reconstructive secondary surgery in patients with large skull bone and other tissue defects and following vascular, brain tumours, and spinal lesions (neuronavigation, biocompatible materials), the stereotactic implantation of deep brain stimulation electrodes for chronic brain stimulation to treat disorders of central motor function with involuntary movements and central deafferentiation pain as well as central functional electrical stimulation for arousal reactions in comatose and vegative state patients. The treatment of spastic functional disorders by intrathecal Baclofen ® application, or, today, by repeated intramuscular injections of Botulinum toxin A and other procedures are recommended.

Phrenic nerve pacing and the urinary bladder stimulation in spinal cord lesions has become part of neurorehabilitation concepts. Since recently vagus nerve stimulation is recommended for the management and rehabilitation in treatment resistant epilepsy. Implantation of neuroprosthesis for VIII cranial nerve stimulation and the FES neurostimulation in para- and tetraplegic patients have shown beneficial results. The development of intelligent networks for restoring the function of central and peripheral motor functional deficits is very promising. The Committee for Neurosurgical Rehabilitation would like to motivate all interested neurosurgeons, physicians and researchers to present and to discuss their ideas and their own results while joining our task force.

Conclusions

All neurorehabilitation measures have one common goal, namely to avoid or to elevate diagnosable or impending damage to the CNS. This means to prevent secondary and tertiary complications by enacting medical, therapeutical measures to simultaneously employ therapeutic programmes with and without special tools – to influence functional, cognitive and behavioural impairments in such a way that every day skill can be regained or in case of communicational and behavioural impairments to use acquisition of skill through brain plasticity in the young and the adult brain. In summery, it is the question of overcoming the social handicap and improving his/her Quality of Life as classified by the 5 dimensional Classification of the WHO ICIDH-2 (morbidity, impairment, activity, participation, and social relationship). In the *spectrum of neurorehabilitation* the neurosurgeon therefore, as we see him/her today, plays an ever more important role, including the establishment and management of the corresponding medical departments and clinics for neurorehabilitation. To describe all these tasks of neurosurgical rehabilitation in detail and to initiate rehabilitation – research efforts, validating therapeutical concepts, and at the same time to elaborate or organise new approaches to quality-assurance are a challenge for neurosurgeons. These are the primary objectives of our Committee.

We sincerely hope that all societies of the WFNS will recognise these opportunities opened up for multidisciplinary-transdisciplinary neurosurgical rehabilitation in view of basic research and clinical application. We also hope that their delegates will join us to implement these in the future. Your are very welcome!

References

1. Boyeson MG, Jones JL (1996) Theoretical mechanisms of brain plasticity and therapeutic implications. In: Horn LJ, Zasler ND (eds) Medical rehabilitation of traumatic brain injury. Hanley and Belfus Inc., Philadelphia, pp 77–102

2. Christensen A-L, Uzzel B (eds) (2000) International Handbook of neuropsychological rehabilitation. Kluwer Academic/Plenum Publishers. New York, Boston, Dordrecht, London, Moscow

3. Diemath HE, Sommerauer J, von Wild KRH (eds) (1996) Brain protection in severe Head injury. W. Zuckschwerdt Verlag, München Bern Wien New York

4. Foerster O (1936) Übungstherapie. In: Bumke O, Foerster O (eds) Handbuch der Neurologie, Bd. 8. Springer, Berlin Heidelberg New York, S316–414

5. Frommelt P, Katzenmeyer F (1999) Zur Geschichte der neurologischen Rehabilitation. In: Frommelt P, Grötzbach H (eds) Neurorehabilitation. Blackwell Wissenschaftsverlag, Berlin Wien, S1–18

6. Gonzáles-Feria L, von Wild KRH, Diemath HE (eds) (2000) Quality management in head injuries care. Servicio Canario de Salud, Santa Cruz de Tenerife

7. Horn LJ, Zasler ND (eds) (1996) Medical rehabilitation of traumatic brain injury. Hanely & Belfus, Philadelphia, USA

8. Kanno T, Okuma I, Yam N (1999) Neurostimulation for arousal of coma. Abstract Book, The 10th Asian Australasian Congress of Neurological Surgery, Lahore, Pakistan, p 118

9. Stein DG (1998) Brain injury and theories of recovery. In: Goldstein LB (ed) Restorative neurology. Futura Publishing Company, Armong, NY, pp 1–34

10. Voss A, von Wild K, and the German Task Force on ENNR (1993) Standards der neurologisch-neurochirurgischen Frührehabilitation. In: von Wild K (ed) Spektrum der Neurorehabilitation W. Zuckschwerdt-Verlag, München Bern Wien New York, S112–120

11. Voss A, von Wild KRH, Prosiegel M (eds) (2000) Qualitätsmanagement in der neurologischen und neurochirurgischen Frührehabilitation. W. Zuckschwerdt Verlag, München Bern Wien New York

12. von Wild KRH, Janzik HH (1993) Zur Begriffsbestimmung: Neurologisch-neurochirurgische Frührehabilitation. In: von Wild K (ed) Spektrum der Neurorehabilitation W. Zuckschwerdt-Verlag, München Bern Wien New York, S109–111

13. von Wild KRH (1999) Are there standards in neurotraumatology? Acta Chir Austriaca 31 [Suppl] 159: 23–27

14. von Wild KRH (ed) (1998) Pathophysiological principles and controversies in neurointensive care. W. Zuckschwerdt-Verlag, München Bern Wien New York

15. von Wild KRH (2000) Perioperative management of severe head injuries in adults. In: Schmidek HH (ed) Operative neurosurgical techniques, 4th edn, vol 1. W. B. Saunders Company, Philadelphia, pp 45–60

16. von Wild KRH (1998/1999) Newsletter, WFNS Neurorehabilitation Committee

Correspondence: Prof. Dr. med Klaus von Wild, Neurochirurgische Klinik, Clemenshospital fmblt, Duesbergweg 124, 48 153 Münster, Germany.

Acta Neurochir (2001) [Suppl] 79: 11–19
© Springer-Verlag 2001

Standards of Neurologic-Neurosurgical Early Rehabilitation – A Concept of the Study Group Neurological-Neurosurgical Early Rehabilitation

E. Ortega-Suhrkamp[1] and **K. R. H. von Wild**[2]

[1] Asklepios Schloßberg-Klinik, Bad, Germany
[2] Clemenshospital Münster, Neurosurgical Department, Münster, Germany

Summary

Neurological neurosurgical early rehabilitation (NNER) is a new important therapeutic link within the spectrum of neurorehabilitation. This concept was formulated by expert opinion of the German Task Force on NNER to define both the structural and process quality of rehabilitation in patients who sustained brain damage with sensory motor, cognitive, and neurobehavioural impairment. NNER is focused on improving higher nervous functions, preventing or treating secondary and tertiary complications and thus to recuse disabilities. This concept is based on interdisciplinary teamwork and needs multidisciplinary cooperation with all specialists involved. The progress of recovery can be measured with the aid of the Coma Remission Scale.

Keywords: Early rehabilitation; traumatic brain injury; standards in neurorehabilitation.

Definition

Early Rehabilitation is an independent concept of diagnostic, rehabilitative, and psychosocial measures. Special emphasis must be attached to ER within the comprehensive chain of rehabilitation due to the severity and complexity of cerebral injuries with secondary disorders of all organic systems.

Similar to the Frauenhofer lines in the solar spectrum, there are also characteristic absorption lines to be found in each brain-injured patient, namely milestones in his individual rehabilitation spectrum that mark his rehabilitation potential, his progress on the road to recovery, and the success attained in his rehabilitation, marks that are found from directly after the time of his brain injury all the way up to his definitive reintegration into society and vocational life or else the determination that there is no rehabilitation potential at all. This process runs along a time axis that can extend over several years, depending on the primary brain injury and the individual rehabilitation potential as well as the intensity and the success of his early and long-term rehabilitation. Neurosurgical-neurological early rehabilitation is an indispensible component of the intensive-care regimen for brain-injured patients.

Our proposal is that in future we speak of a spectrum of neurologico-neurosurgical rehabilitation that can be used to describe the temporal dynamicity of measures for early and long-term rehabilitation for the individual patient.

In the continuous solar spectrum, then according to the distribution of intensities of differing wavelengths, the colours continuously mingle with each other, from blue-violet via blue, green, yellow, and orange to yellow-red, and the object under investigation shows characteristic absorption lines, the so-called Frauenhofer lines (Fig. 1).

Much in the same way, in the continuous, fluctuating spectrum of neurologico-neurosurgical rehabilitation, the various rehabilitation measures – oriented solely towards the functional status of the brain-injured patient at any given time – glide smoothly from the early-rehabilitation phase into the long-term rehabilitation. In this regard, early-rehab measures first accompany the acute therapy – for example early on during the intensive-care phase – and later on, when the patient's vigilance has improved, to gradually assume the leading role in the therapeutic concept, all the way up to the transfer to an early-rehabilitation facility. This facility can be part of a central hospital, but also of a rehabilitation clinic. The long-term rehabilitation follows on from this seamlessly.

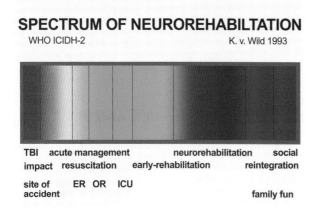

SPECTRUM OF NEUROREHABILTATION
WHO ICIDH-2   K. v. Wild 1993

TBI   acute management   neurorehabilitation   social
impact   resuscitation   early-rehabilitation   reintegration

site of   ER OR ICU
accident   family fun

Fig. 1. Spectrum of neurologico-neurosurgical rehabilitation. The spectrum of neurological-neurosurgical rehabilitation. By analogy to the solar spectrum with the Frauenhofer lines, the figure shows the continuous, fluctuating transition over time (t) of the individual rehab measures, starting with the early-rehabilitation phase and ending with the reintegration of the patient into vocational life and society after successful long-term rehabilitation. This spectrum is characteristic for each individual patient, and is dependent on the remaining plasticity and the rehabilitation potential

To meet the requirements, ER therapy needs more staff than any other form of rehabilitation, and is therefore very costly and also demands special room facilities. The position of ER within the rehabilitation chain does not correspond to the term "Phase 1b" used by vocational cooperatives. This concept refers to patients with various degrees of disorders, all the way to the complete loss of consciousness or in a permanent vegetative state. Further symptoms of the syndrome are pronounced vegetative disorders with absence of the so-called protective reflexes of the brain stem, resulting in vital threat. Often there is a massive spastic increase of muscle tone that may in turn lead to joint contractures. Lacking postural reflexes prohibit head and body control, so that even sitting in a wheelchair becomes difficult. The result is absolute helplessness. Brain injuries in accident injured patients are frequently combined with complicated fractures and further trauma-dependent damage of secondary organic systems (combined traumatic brain injury), a feature that complicates therapy and increases the cost of treatment.

Another group are patients *in a transitional syndrome of confusion (Durchgangssyndrom)*, which is characterized by marked restlessness, local, time, and situative disorientation, linked with partly depressive, partly aggressive expression, and more or less distinct motion disturbances.

The most severe brain damage might be determined by: trauma, cerebral circulation problems and hemorrhage, intoxication, hypoxia, inflammation, tumor etc. According to our understanding, neurologic-neurosurgical ER consists of comprehensive, individual, and interdisciplinary therapy measures that should be enacted as soon as possible to achieve the following *objectives*:

1. To support and/or enhance the course of spontaneous remission
2. To maximize the existing rehabilitation potential by promoting brain plasticity and to counteract undesirable developments
3. To avoid secondary damage
4. To recognize/diagnose and eliminate secondary damage (e.g. hydrocephalus)
5. To reduce and avoid tertiary damage (e.g. chronic infections, contractures, pressure sores, osteoporosis).

Admission criteria: Severely brain-injured patients are eligible for admission to the ER department provided they are

– no longer on the ventilator
– sufficiently stable in terms of circulation
– without increased intracranial pressure, and
– not suffering from severe infection.

Central venous catheters, partial parenteral application (PPN), tracheostoma, and suprapubic catheter do not constitute exclusion criteria.

As a rule, exclusion criteria include progressive cerebral diseases such as M. Alzheimer, Chorea Huntington.

The admission of each individual patient is decided by the ER department concerned. The initiation of ER and its duration can be determined only considering each individual course. ER therapy should not be considered as permanent therapy. During the course of therapy, a decision must be met regarding the transfer of the patient; this might be directly into a further rehabilitation clinic, into a long-term therapeutic nursing home, or into home care – the option of intermittent therapy is also open.

Most important *criteria to cut off* ER:

– partial mobilization of the patient (also in wheelchair)
– improvement of disturbed vegetative function (bladder, bowel)

– re-established communication skills
– improved cognitive functions
– obeying simple orders must be possible, i.e. active cooperation in simple actions
– diminishing behavioral problems.

In children and young people there are admission, discharge, and duration criteria that take the special situation of this patient group into account.

Staffing of an Early Rehabilitation Department

The staffing requirement is calculated for a department of 15–20 beds provided that the (therapeutic) team works interdisciplinary and in a patient-centered mode. If added to an existing department, staffing and room programs need to be adapted. Such a department ought to be headed by a neurologist or neurosurgeon, or in the case of children and young people by a neuropediatrician. Continuing training and experience in neurological rehabilitation should be prerequisites.

Individual deviations might be necessary according to regional conditions in acute top-level care clinics or neurological rehabilitation centers and dependent on the severity and complexity of the damage as well as on the age of the neurological patient. This is especially relevant to departments treating children and adolescents.

Teamwork

The prime objective of the entire team is to support the patient sensomotorically, cognitively, and socially by utilizing the regeneration ability and plasticity of

Table 1. *Staff Requirement of an ER Department (Calculated for 15–20 Beds)*

Medical physicians	1/1/2
For following staff requirements the ratio of therapist to patients is given:	
Psychologist	1:15
Nurses	1:0.4–0.75
Speech therapy	1:7,5
Physiotherapy	1:15
Occupational therapy	1:4 to 1:5
Social services	1:15
Pedagogist service	1:7.5
Additional personnel: 1 technical assistant for electrophysiological diagnostic procedures,	
1 secretary,	
1.5 ward assistants if not covered by central services	

the brain, as long as is necessary to transgress from the acute stage into a progressive remission stage.

According to our experience and observations, about 70% of the patients can be saved from the most severe handicap by adequate therapy. This goal can be reached only with all professionals working on and with the patient, not only in the proficiency-centered fashion, but also in interdisciplinary cooperation within the team. One therapist should help the patient continuously to understand his surroundings, which may appear foreign and even frightening to him. The cooperation of all the various professionals involved optimizes the intensive care and support for the patient to be activated. Qualification, experience, and psychophysical resistance are prerequisites for all team workers to be up to the task. Regular intern and, if necessary, extern postgraduate education for all professionals specifically as well as interdisciplinary education is essential. In order for the team to hold their ground under this strenuous workload, case-specific team supervision should ideally be included in intern education. Such institutional team supervision ought to be conducted by an external clinically experienced supervisor. In regular intervals the progress of rehabilitation is assessed by the team members (best functional result) with the aid of the Coma Remission Scale (Table 4a+b).

Responsibility of Medical Services

Besides the usual medical routine the doctor has to supervise and to coordinate therapies in ER. The therapeutic course is decided on in cooperation with all therapists and nurses. The doctor conducts patient-specific team conferences and decides on how to continue in all cases of doubt. In order to work in a well-coordinated and integrational fashion within the team, the doctor ought to have practical education in all the relevant therapeutic areas.

Psychological Services

The special task of the psychologist is the exact behavioral observation of the patient. This includes also continuous process observation in order to rapidly adapt therapies to all changes in the situation. Psychosocial work ranges from single- and group-therapeutic talks on coping strategies and crisis intervention with patients to trauma-induced conflict- and problem-solving with the involved family. They need to cope

with the severe illness and often many months of therapy of the patient in ER – of course, at the beginning
there is more work with the family than with the
patient. Neuropsychological diagnosis is done as soon
as the patient has gained a certain degree of stress
tolerance and is able to cooperate, and has started to
understand his illness. It is not possible to pin down,
differentiate, and to specifically treat cognitive deficiencies until this stage is reached.

Nursing Services

Nursing services occupy a special role in ER. They
are responsible for the care of severely ill patients who
are on the ward for many months. Nursing staff is integrated within the therapeutic team. Besides basic and
specialized nursing including intensive care measures
of neurology, neurosurgery, and psychiatry, an important contribution of their work is the activating
part of nursing (stimulation, activation, positioning,
mobilization, etc.).

In close cooperation with other therapists the nurses
adapt their therapeutic task into everyday care for the
patient.

Physiotherapeutic Services

The sooner careful, systematic motoric therapy is
started, the more favourable progress will be. Careful
in this sense means enacting treatment as painlessly as
possible and influencing progress favorably through
special stimulation (e.g. vestibulary). First of all patients ought to be positioned opposite to their "pattern", then therapeutic influence of spasticity and motoric restlessness ought to have priority. Later holding
reactions are started and finally voluntary movements
are promoted. Contractures should be avoided and
existing contractures reduced.

Occupational Therapy Services

The individual priorities are set on the basis of admission findings. These may be:

– early promotion; basal stimulation, facio-oral therapy, sensomotoric integration
– motor-functional training
– treatment of perception disorders: tactile, proprio-
  receptive, vestibulary, visual-acoustic, gustatory,
  and olfactory

– communication
– music therapy
– activity of daily life training
– testing of auxiliary parts and furnishing
– home care visit.

Speech Therapist Services

The therapeutic interventions in speech and swallowing have the following emphasis:

– reduction of pathological oral reflex activity
– basal stimulation of muscles involved in speech and
  swallowing
– mobilizing techniques to stimulate very first movements
– specific mobility training to stimulate speech functions and food intake
– general stimulation of communication
– special diagnosis and speech-systematic as well as
  communicative therapy (following improvement of
  cognitive function).

Social Services

Social services with rehabilitation counselling has
the task of psychosocial counselling and care of the
patient or/and the family involved, for example:

– counselling in economic problems, explaining of
  special pension funds, support in problems with insurance and administrative bodies,
– establishing or re-establishing of contact to friends
  and neighbours.

(Therapeutic) Pedagogist Services

Their task involves:

– early promotion of the coma patient through improvement of vigilance and attention by stimulating
  all perceptive channels,
– functional training and as soon as possible intellec-
  tual and cognitive training on a pedagogic-didactic
  foundation,
– re-establishment of group and communication ability,
– influencing behaviour disorders through behaviour
  therapy-oriented training, avoiding putting too
  great or too small strain on the patient.

Room Program

So far there is no sufficient experience to introduce an obligatory room program. In principle it is safe to assume that an ER department requires a very large room capacity. This is justified by the great variety of treatment forms in the department itself, the high number of staff needed, the support for all the family involved, and last but not least by the great amount of individual nursing material needed for each patient.

The following numbers refer to a department of 15 beds in a newly erected building and must be adapted accordingly if extended.

Table 2. *Therapy Room Capacity*

Physiotherapy
Occupational therapy
Music therapy
Language therapy
Speech therapy
Hydrotherapy
Psychologist
Medical physician
Group activity room
Lounge for next-of-kin
Storage room
Neurophysiological laboratory
Secretary's office
Social services
Pedagogic staff
Nursing services
In addition: 30% floor space and lounge area for staff, also a room for casting

Table 3. *Equipment of an ER Department (Calculated for 15–20 Beds)*

11	Special beds for cardiac patients, including bedside table
4	Special beds to prevent pressure sores, e.g. air-cushion bed plus bedside tables
4	Special beds to enable complete upright position in bed
2	Patient-transfer and shower systems
3–5	Wheelchairs
2	Transfer systems for lifting patients
3	Shower wheelchairs
4	Patient-monitoring systems for ECG, EEG, EVP (central monitor system)
5	Defibrillator
3–6	Microcomputers
1	Diagnostic area for EEG and EVP
2	Diagnostic area for EMG and Doppler
3	Ventilator (with endoscope)
4	Mobile x-ray machine
5	Biochemical emergency laboratory
CCT (and MRT) readily available or within 15 minutes transport in very close locality	

Rooms for the patients: The rooms for the patients ought to be furnished in a flexible way so as to allow up to four patients per room. In any case single bedrooms as well as twin bedrooms should also be available. The rooms ought to be of sufficient size to permit the treatment of the patient in his own room in the very early stage.

Single bedrooms ought to be 20 m^2 in size, twin bedrooms 30 m^2. Bathroom units are not included.

Cooperation with Next-of-Kin

According to up-to-date experience, the patient's next-of-kin should be included in the treatment and caring for the patient. Indications are:

– The next-of-kin know the personal structure of the patient from the time before the event, a feature that is prerequisite for individual treatment.
– The next-of-kin usually make more detailed observations than do the clinic staff and often are the first to register conscious reactions of the coma patient.
– The next-of-kin are trusted by the patient and especially in the early stage are therefore able to calm the disoriented and confused patient, thus helping to avoid or reduce vegetative disregulation.
– The next-of-kin accompany frightened patients to their therapy sessions and help in the stimulation process by taking care of various everyday life activities.

We do not consider it wise to encourage 24-hour care by the next-of-kin. This rapidly leads to stress for the patient as well as for the family concerned apart from impeding on the relationship with the team of therapists, which is important for treatment. The state of illness often puts undue stress on the family. Intensive talks with the doctor and psychologist are necessary to help understand the illness and the various remission stages. It is only through understanding the actual situation of the severely ill patient that the family will be able to avoid putting strain on the patient and aggravating his state of health further still. Psychotherapeutic talks must help to work on fear, uncertainty, and grieving reactions of the family. The objective of these discussions is the establishment of the best possible foundation of cooperation between the patient's next-of-kin and team members in order to avoid mutual unfair reproaches and blaming each other. These talks can take place individually as well as in the group setting. In addition there ought to be regular gatherings of families concerned to meet up with representatives of all parts of the therapeutic team. Besides the exchange of general information, therapists may introduce the next-of-kin to their specific part of activity, give instructions on how to stimulate the patient or offer self-experience experiments.

Regional Supply

An overall network of ER departments is necessary, ideally being based at acute-care hospitals or suitable rehabilitation centers. Sufficient regional supply is defined for the admission area of the patient group to cover no more than 150–200 km. In case of necessary involvement of the family, they should be able to get to the treatment facility within one to two hours. In addition it is wise to establish close cooperation between the acute-care clinic and the neurological ER department. Medical services of the ER department might advise colleagues as well as therapists and nurses in difficult cases or long waiting lists on further therapeutic course until the patient is transferred to ER. Also very first talks with the family might start at the acute care clinic.

Conclusions

The concept of neurologic-neurosurgical early rehabilitation requires everyone involved to reorient their attitudes to this area, away from the separation into curative medicine and rehabilitation that has been the case in the past with its inherent classification of disorders into phases, and instead towards a concept that is not fraught by interface problems as demanded by a holistic approach to neurorehabilitation.

Institution

Neurological neurosurgical early rehabilitation is a very important link in the chain of rehabilitation measures (Spectrum on Neurorehabilitation). A network of ER departments in acute-care hospitals and rehabilitation centres should be established.

In acute-care hospitals neurosurgical, neurological, and neuroradiological departments as well as intensive care need to be provided.

For rehabilitation clinics essential: neurosurgical, neurological, and neuroradiological departments must

be available within 15–20 minutes. Close cooperation must be established with medical services of the areas in accident surgery, eye, ENT, and internal medicine.

Special room and staffing capacity are prerequisites. A unit of 20 beds with single and twin bedrooms appears the most advisable, taking into account the calculated staffing situation there should be no fewer than 15 beds for adults and 10 beds for children and young people.

Concerning the establishment of an ER department within the acute-care hospital, the direct transfer of the patient into a neurological rehabilitation clinic must be ensured.

Demand

Various authors have determined the demand for neurological ER departments. However, within the study group there are serious reservations that an overcapacity might develop in the near future. The number of clinics planned from the sociopolitical viewpoint should be critically assessed and corrected accordingly on a regular basis. In the best interest of the patient, the demanded high standard of care ought to be secured and developed further still by means of continuous quality management.

Research

Research in neurological ER demands a close intermeshing of basic research and clinical practice. Since research cannot be financed through nursing and treatment fees, a third financial source must be made available.

Priorities might be:

- The development and critical scrutiny of coma-stimulation therapies
- Critical testing of pharmacological treatment for brain protection
- Investigation of brain metabolism and cerebral circulation of severely brain damaged patients during the acute stage and the progressive course
- Evaluation of therapies used up to now
- Development and assessment of evaluation scales for benchmarking
- Long-term studies for the prognosis and outcome of brain damage, in single-case studies and on an epidemiological scale.

Table 4a Items (Front)

Coma Remission Scale (CRS)

GERMAN TASK FORCE ON

Neurological-Neurosurgical
Early Rehabilitation 1993 (13)

Patient name:

Date:	
Investigator (initials):	

1. Arousability/attention (to any stimulus)

Attention span for 1 minute or longer	5	
Attention remains on stimulus (longer than 5 sec)	4	
Turning towards a stimulus	3	
Spontaneous eye opening	2	
Eye opening in response to pain	1	
None	0	

2. Motoric response (minus 6 points from max. attainable sum if tetraplegic)

Spontaneous grasping (also from prone position)	6	
Localized movement in response to pain	5	
Body posture recognizable	4	
Unspecific movement in response to pain (vegetative or spastic pattern)	3	
Flexion in response to pain	2	
Extension in response to pain	1	
None	0	

3. Response to acoustic stimuli (e.g. clicker) (minus 3 points from max. attainable sum if deaf)

Recognizes a well-acquainted voice, music, etc.	3	
Eye opening, turning of head, perhaps smiling	2	
Vegetative reaction (startle)	1	
None	0	

4. Response to visual stimuli (minus 4 points from max. attainable sum if blind)

Recognizes pictures, persons, objects	4	
Follows pictures, persons, objects	3	

Table 4a+b. *Continued*

Table 4a Items (Front)

Fixates on pictures, persons, objects	2	
Occasional, random eye movements	1	
None	0	

5. Response to tactile stimuli

Recognizes by touching/feeling	3	
Spontaneous, targeted grasping (if blind), albeit without comprehension of sense	2	
Only vegetative response to passive touching	1	
None	0	

6. Auditory response (tracheostoma = 3 if lips can be heard to utter guttural sounds/seen to mime "letters")

At least one understandably articulated word	3	
Unintelligible (unarticulated) sounds	2	
Groaning, screaming, coughing (emotional, vegetatively tinged)	1	
No phonetics/articulation audible/recognizable	0	

Sum score:		
Max. Attainable score (of 24) for this patient		

Table 4b Guidance (Back)

1. Arousability/attention

    5 pts: Patient can direct his/her attention towards an interesting stimulus for at least 1 minute (perceivable by vision, hearing, or touching; stimulus: persons, objects, noises, music, voices, etc.) without being diverted by secondary stimuli.

    4 pts: Attention fixed to a stimulus for a discernible moment (fixation with the eyes, grasping, and feeling or "pricking up of ears"); patient is, however, easily diverted or "switches off".

    3 pts: Patient turns to source of stimulus by moving eyes, head, or body; patient follows moving objects. Vegetative reactions should also be observed (patient capable only of vegetative reaction).

    2 pts: Spontaneous opening of eyes without any external stimulus, e.g. in connection with a sleep-waking-state rhythm.

2. Motoric response

    6 pts: Patient spontaneously grasps hold of held-out everyday objects (only if patient's vision function is intact, otherwise lay object on back of patient's hand) OR patient able to respond to such gestures with an invitational character only with a delay or inconsistently, yet adequately, due to paralysis or contraction.

    Note regarding the following items (use of pain stimuli):

        The pain stimuli must be applied to the various limbs and to the body trunk, since there may be regional stimulus-perception impairments; pain stimuli can take the form e.g. of a gentle twisting pinch of a fold of skin, pressure applied to a fingernail fold, tickling of the nose.

    5 pts: Patient responds to pain stimuli defensively after localization, by a targeted and adequate measure, e.g. pushing away, sweeping motions of the hand, etc.

    4 pts: The patient should be seated upright: tests for the sense of balance and/or posture by slight pushes applied to the body (corrective movements of trunk or extremities).

    3 pts: Untargeted withdrawal from pain stimulus or merely vegetative reactions (tachycardia, tachypnea, agitation) or increase of spastic pattern.

    2 pts: Strong, hardly resolvable flexion, especially in the arms/elbows. Legs may stretch out.

    1 pt: Typical "decerebrate rigidity" with spastic extension of all extremities, in many cases opisthotonus (dorsal overextension/hyperlordosis).

Table 4a+b. *Continued*

Table 4b Guidance (Back)

3. *Response to acoustic stimuli (tests as a rule to be carried out beyond patient's field of vision!)*
   3 pts: Patient can recognize voices or music, i.e. he/she is able either to name the stimulus or to react in a differentiated manner (e.g. to certain pieces of music or persons with pleasure or defensively).
   2 pts: Patient only opens eyes, fixates or turns to source of stimulus with his/her head, in some cases accompanied by emotional expressions such as smiling, crying, ...
   1 pt: Rise in pulse and/or blood pressure, perspiration or agitation, excessive twitching of the body, slight triggering of eye blinking.
   Note: Similar to the procedures applied when testing the motoric responsiveness by the application of pain stimuli, the use of a clicker held directly next to each of the patient's ears (bilateral testing) suggests itself as the relatively strongest non-pain-involving stimulus for items 1 and 2; if the response is positive, the patient can be assumed to still be in possession of his/her hearing and the stimuli can be made more manifold.

4. *Response to visual stimuli (must be presented without speaking or any other form of comment)*
   4 pts: Patient recognizes pictures, objects, portraits of familiar persons.
   3 pts: Follows pictures etc. with the eyes without any sign of recognition or questioning, inconsistent recognition.
   2 pts: Fixates moving pictures or objects without being able to follow them properly, or when picture/object moves outside patient's field of vision patient makes no attempt to keep track.

5. *Response to tactile stimuli*
   3 pts: Patient capable of feeling and recognizing objects, hands of other persons, etc. even if his/her sense of vision is absent and the objects must be placed on the skin/in the hands; adequate response to stimuli in the area of the mouth/face (edible/inedible, e.g. response to a kiss).
   2 pts: Touches, feels, and grasps targetedly, but without an adequate reaction.
   1 pt: Unspecific response to stroking and touch (vegetative signs such as agitation, raised pulse).

6. *Auditory response*
   3 pts: Patient is capable of expressing an intelligible word, even if this is not related to the context or situation. Names also count as words here.
   2 pts: Patient utters unintelligible sounds, e.g. slurred, also repetition of syllables or similar ("ma-ma", "au", ...).

Total score: In the event that certain channels of sense or motor systems are completely absent ("blind", "deaf", "plegic"), the point scores of the respective category must be subtracted from the maximum attainable score, e.g. 12/21 points instead of 12/24 points.

Reference

1. Voss A, von Wild, KRH, Prosiegel M (eds) (2000) Qualitätsmanagement in der neurologischen und neurochirurgischen Frührehabilitation. W. Zuckschwerdt-Verlag, München Bern Wien New York

Correspondence: E. Ortega-Suhrkamp, Asklepios Schloßberg-Klinik, Frankfurter Straße 33, D-64732 Bad, Germany.

Acta Neurochir (2001) [Suppl] 79: 21–23

Early Rehabilitative Concepts in Therapy of the Comatose Brain Injured Patients

M. Lippert-Grüner, C. Wedekind, R.-I. Ernestus, and **N. Klug**

Klinik für Allgemeine Neurochirurgie, der Universität zu Köln, Köln, Germany

Summary

Objectives. To evaluate the changes of vegetative parameters and behavioural assessment in comatous patients after severe brain injury during the Multimodal-Early-Onset-Stimulation (MEOS) in early rehabilitation.

Material and Methods. We studied 16 predominantly male (3:1) patients, age mean 43.6 (16–77) years. Mean coma duration was 22.2 (8–41) days, therapy duration (MEOS) 9.8 (1–30) days. The initial GCS was 6.6 (3–9), KRS 5.3 (0–15). Including criteria for therapy: Severe head trauma, coma for at least 48 hours (GCS < 8), vegetative stability, normal intracranial pressure, abandon of mechanical ventilation, sedation and severe infections. MEOS was finished in achieving GCS > 9, follow-up investigations were made after 2 years.

Results. We identified significant changes in two vegetative parameters (heart/respiratory frequencies), even in deep coma (GCS 3–4). Most significant changes were caused by tactile and acoustic stimulation. Standardized behavioural assessment turned out to be particularly advisable in cases of medium coma (GCS 5–7). Stimulation of tactile and acoustic senses resulted mainly in mimical, head and eye movements. Follow-up was possible in 14 patients: One remained in a vegetative state (GOS 2), two exhibited severe neurologic/neuropsychologic deficits, depending on care (GOS 3), six substained major functional deficits (GOS 4), at though they were able to perform the tasks of daily life on their own, three patients reached GOS 5. Two returned to their former jobs.

Discussion and Conclusion. The present results indicate that stimulation therapy should be based on a close observation of patterns of behaviour, and, at least in deep coma stages, involve the registration of vegetative parameters. It may be sensitive to identify parameters predicting a favourable or unfavourable outcome. Preliminary data seem to support the hypothesis that the absence of any response to external stimuli is indicative of an unfavourable outcome.

Keywords: Early neurorehabilitation; sensory stimulation; traumatic coma.

Introduction

Early rehabilitation is an integrated interdisciplinary therapy, which starts early and proceeds continuously with changing points of interest. Its aim is to support spontaneous recovery, to reduce the risk of early and late complications, and to make intensive use of the brain's own rehabilitative ability and plasticity.

At present, it has not been possible to make a reliable prognosis about the recovery from the "vegetative posttraumatic state", not even on the basis of clinical data or electrophysiologic data such as evoked potentials. Consequently, other electrophysiologic examinations like event-related potentials or the analysis of changes in the EEG-spectre are increasingly used to detect covert reactions to external stimuli. Until now, this diagnosis of sensory or cognitive capacities in comatose patients or patients with reduced consciousness has proven to be very difficult. Since patients appear to react to stimuli from their surroundings, an observation which is often reported by close relatives, it is believed that to a certain extent comatose patients are able to process external stimuli. Reuter *et al.* (1989) showed that slow cortical potentials can be used to characterize mental functions as well as to assess comatose patients' chances of recovery.

In the literature, there is no satisfactory answer to the question whether further specific measures can enhance to the healing process and accelerate recovery from coma [1, 6]. Experiments carried out on animals have disclosed the possibility of changing patterns of neuronal activation by means of external influences like auditory, tactile, or visual stimulation [5]. Over the last few years sensory stimulation has played an increasingly important role in early rehabilitation therapy.

Patients and Methods

We report on a regime of multimodal stimulation performed in comatose patients during early rehabilitation at a neurosurgical intensive care unit. Patients who have been comatous for more than 48 hours after trauma were selected for this therapy.

The present study, which was carried out over a period of two years, focuses on 89 patients aged 16–65 years suffering from severe brain injury. Sixteen of them (mean Age: 43.6 years) qualified for multimodal-early-onset-stimulation-therapy (MEOS), which lasted for an average of 9.8 (range 1–30) days. The patients received early rehabilitation treatment at the neurosurgical intensive care unit for an average time period of 27.9 days. The mean Glasgow Coma Score (GCS) at the beginning of the stimulation therapy was 6.56 (range 3–9).

The stimulation therapy consists of auditory, tactile, olfactory, gustatory and kinesthetic procedures, administered daily in two units of one hour each.

Special restrictions have to be made concerning frequency and intensity of sensory stimulation in order to avoid overly straining the injured brain. Controlled stimulation therapy should include low noise levels and adequate intervals between stimulation and medical and nursing activities. Furthermore, the patient's notion of time should be supported by alternating phases of activity and intervals without therapy. Rather than following a static pattern, stimulation units are based on dialogue answers and the actual level of function achieved in the several sections.

The so-called dialogue answers to stimulation only appear at changes of vegetative parameters in the coma patient. Such reactions are monitored during the whole stimulation phase by means of a feedback for system recording and continuous registration of heart rate and respiration rate and galvanic skin response, including the possibility of direct graphical reproduction. These electrophysiological data were recorded and analyzed with the Paron-biofeedback device (PAR Elektronik GmbH) and the VITAPORT system developed at Cologne University. The VITAPORT system allows the co-registration of EEG and EMG.

The observation of the patient's behaviour becomes increasingly important as coma depth decreases. A standardized behavioural assessment protocol was developed during the first stages of the examinations on the basis of the KRS (Koma-Remissions-Scale), which also focuses on vegetative changes. The patient's most frequent reactions were clarified into mimic reactions, vocal utterings, arousability/attentiveness, motor reactions and vegetative changes.

Results and Conclusions

Clinical observations of the patients under stimulation revealed that changes in vegetative parameters (e.g. in changes of the heart rate and respiration rate) precede any visible behavioral change. To prove whether these changes differ from baseline without stimulation, a 10 minute baseline before stimulation and every 10 minutes between the stimulation sessions (A-B-A design) was recorded.

We were able to identify changes in the vegetative parameters (heart rate and respiration rate) of our patients, even those in deep coma (GCS 3–4). Figure 1 displays the monitoring of a multimodal stimulation therapy administered to a 38-year old patient, a therapy which was begun on the 4th posttraumatic day. At that time, the GCS reached 4 points. During stimulation, the heart rate showed significant changes, especially during tactile stimulation.

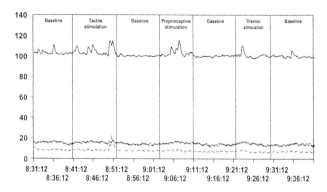

Fig. 1. Stimulation of D.A., a 38-year old patient, as soon as four days after he sustained severe brain injury (GSC 4) does cause observable stimulation-dependent changes in the heart rate (highest line)

The most important changes were found during tactile and acoustic stimulation. Standardized behavioural assessment turned out to be particularly advisable in cases with GCS 5–6. Again, a stimulation of the tactile and acoustic senses resulted mainly in head and eye movements.

Two years later, 14 patients were reexamined, whilst two patients were prevented from attending the examination by structural problems. One of the patients examined had remained in a vegetative state (GOS 2), two suffered from severe neurological and neuropsychological deficits and were dependent on care (GOS 3), six exhibited from functional deficiencies, though they did perform the tasks of daily life on their own (GOS 4), and three had a GOS of 5. Two of these had been able to return to their old jobs.

It seems important to identify parameters predicting a favorable outcome in non-responding comatose patients during diagnostic stimulation. At present, the number of observations available is still too small to provide a final answer to this question, and the follow-up is too short to determine the usefulness of this diagnostic approach. Preliminary data seem to support the hypothesis that the absence of any response to external stimuli is indicative of an unfavorable outcome. However, we cannot infer a good prognosis from patients' capacity to give vegetative responses.

References

1. Kater KM (1989) Response of head-injured patients to sensory stimulation. Western J Nurs Res 11(1): 20–33
2. Mitchell S, Bradley VA, Welch JL, Britton PG (1990) Coma arousal procedure: therapeutic intervention in the treatment of head injury. Brain Injury 4(3): 273–279

3. Pierce JP, Lyle DM, Quine S, Evans NJ, Morris J, Fearnside MR (1990) The effectiveness of coma arousal intervention. Brain Injury 4(2): 191–197

4. Reuter BM, Linke DB, Kurthen M (1989) Cognitive processes in comatose patients? A brain mapping study using P 300. Arch Psychol 141(3): 155–173

5. Rosenzweig MR (1980) Animal models for effects of brain lesions and for rehabilitation. In: Bach-y-Rita P (ed) Recovery of function. Theoretical considerations for brain injury rehabilitation. University Park Press, Baltimore, pp 127–172.

6. Schreiber P, Mai N (1990) Überlegung zur spezifischen Rehabilitation bei Patienten mit schwerem Schädel-Hirn-Trauma. Rehabilitation 29: 238–241

Correspondence: Dr. M. Lippert-Grüner, Klinik für Allgemeine Neurochirurgie, der Universität zu Köln, Köln, Germany.

Acta Neurochir (2001) [Suppl] 79: 25–29

Incidence and Management of Complications During Posttraumatic Early Rehabilitation

B. Hoffmann and **K. R. H. von Wild**

Clemenshospital Münster, Neurosurgical Department, Münster, Germany

Summary

Early rehabilitation after traumatic brain injury has become a worldwide accepted interface between intensive care medicine and rehabilitation to aim for a better functional outcome of the surviving patients. So each chain can only be as strong as its weakest link, and there is still need for well defined quality standards depending on the medical demands during this period of treatment. Hence we were interested in quantifying the complications occurring until discharge to further rehabilitation with special regard on severe physical handicaps and organ failure necessitating surgical or intensive care therapy. Our results demonstrate that early rehabilitation is a part of intensive care medicine with enhanced approaches to preserve rehabilitation potential of the brain and for coma stimulation.

Keywords: Complications; early rehabilitation; posttraumatic coma.

Introduction

Modern neurotraumatology is a very dynamic faculty of neurosurgery facing a physical catastrophe of 30% of the patients still dying after brain injury [1]. On the other hand promising approaches [2] may offer possibilities for more effective ICP control to minimize mortality as well as improvement of life quality after successful operation, intensie care treatment, and rehabilitation. Early rehabilitation today is accepted worldwide to be a necessary interface between the acute stage and rehabilitation still providing all invasive and non-invasive procedures to intervene on the occasion of complications striking the patient after discharge from the ICU. So early rehabilitation implies subtle neuromonitoring on the one hand and full impact of neurosurgical intensive care medicine on the other. So we try hard to begin coma stimulation therapies as early as possible after vital stabilization of the patient; success of early rehabilitation will also depend on the control of complications.

Patients and Methods

We performed a retrospective analysis on 252 consecutive TBI patients. The population and age pyramid corresponds to the common studies on epidemiology [3]. There was no preselection of patients, neither at admission in the emergency nor later at the threshold between ICU and the Early Rehabilitation Unit. So the rehabilitation team was completely integrated in the programme of work of the neurosurgical department. There is no lack of information up to the end of early rehabilitation and discharge to the rehabilitation hospital. The diagnostical battery is identical to the invasive and non-invasive multimodal monitoring on our ICU (Table 1) so that online diagnosis of intercurring insults is guaranteed.

Results

Of the total of 252 patients 68% belonged to the initial GCS 3–8, 22% to GCS 9–12 and 10% to GCS 13–15. Mean duration of ICU treatment was 7,2 days, mean duration of early rehabilitation 51 days (range of 4–388 days). In this group we saw complications in 134 of the 252 patients. CNS/neurosurgical complications occurred in 27% of the patients, and 27% suffered also from one or more pulmonal complications. The cardiovascular system has been afflicted in 19% of the

Table 1. *Diagnostic Battery for Neurotraumatological ICU and Early Rehabilitation Unit*

Invasive and non-invasive hemodynamic monitoring
ICP (Parenchyma/ventricular)
Monitoring of oxygenation
SaO_2 (peripheral)
RSO_2 (NIRS)
$PtiO_2$ (Licox® system)
EEG, EVOP (Digitally recorded and saved)
Continuous transcranial Doppler sonography

ICP Intracranial pressure, *NIRS* near infrared spectroscopy, *PtiO₂* cerebral oxygen tissue partial pressure.

Table 2. *Neurosurgical Secondary Operations*

Cranioplasty (autologuous/alloplastic)	38
Ventricular-peritoneal-shunt	20
Subdural efffusions, burrhole	9
Shuntrevision, mechanical failure	8
Revision of the frontal skull base	4
CSF fistula	2
Reconstruction of the orbital roof	2
Subdural hematoma, craniotomy, evacuation	4
CSF fistula	3
CSDH, burrhole/craniotomy	3
Brain abscess	2
Neurolysis	2
Median nerve	1
Ulnar nerve	1
Ruptured aneurysm (Clip dislocation)	1
Carotid-cavernosus-fistula	1
Epidural hematoma, craniotomy, evacuation	1
Growing contusion, craniotomy, evacuation	1
Externa ventriculostomy	1
Flap revision	1

Table 3. *GOS Outcome after Intensive Care and Early Rehabilitation Treatment*

GOS 1	6%
GOS 2	6%
GOS 3	47%
GOS 4	24%
GOS 5	18%

cases, metabolic decompensation has been observed in 18%, abdominal complications in 9% of the total.

This means we performed 98 neurosurgical secondary operations in 71 patients, 23% of them needing more than one operation. Twenty-six percent of the procedures took place in the first 10 days of early rehabilitation, 71% between days 1 and 30. The surgical procedures represented a wide range of neurosurgical interventions (Table 2).

Eighty-nine of the patients needed mechanical support of breathing between 4 days and 3 months, 8 patients needed controlled ventilation up to 72 hours. Most cases (68) of respiratory failure referred to aspiration because of neurogenic swallowing disorders with or without impaired consciousness. Thirty-one patients showed severe mucostasis with partial obliteration of main bronchi, 71 patients dystelectasis, 21 patients pneumonia and 2 patients thromboembolism with fatal course in both cases. Fibreoptic bronchoscopy from diagnostical or therapeutical reasons was performed in 71 of the cases.

Thirty patients were admitted with signs of cardial decompensation or developed heart insufficiency during the early rehabilitation treatment and mobilization. Five patients showed severe reduction of heart minute volume due to catecholamine support. Instable coronary disease showed 10 of the patients, one 74 year old patient suffered infarction following pharmacological stimulation. 30 cases of arrhythmia and 91 cases of arterial hypertension could be controlled medically without events.

The most common metabolic problem after reduction of glucose tolerance (42 cases) was CSWS (cerebral salt wasting syndrome) in 12 cases. Diabetes insipidus was observed in 11 patients. Hypocortisolism and hypothyreoidism occurred in 7 cases each.

The main problem in abdominal organs was diarrhea (18 patients). Pseudomembranous enterocolitis with proof of Clostridium difficile was diagnosed in 4 patients, 4 cases could be correlated with nutrition, 1 case followed exocrinic failure of the pancreas, 2 cases resulted from virus infections, for the rest a clear diagnosis could not be found. Six patients suffered from acute pancreatitis from papillospasm, all these cases recovered without persisting handicaps. Hemorrhagic gastritis occurred in 4 patients, Ulcus ventriculi in 3 cases and colon perforation in 2 patients with need for laparotomy.

Since we were interested only in those patients who survived up to the beginning of early rehabilitation, we observed only 6% in the GOS 1 group. Also 6% of the patients were demitted to further rehabilitation on GOS 2, 47% on GOS 3, 24% on GOS 4 and 18% on GOS 5 (Table 3). All of the patients with a favourable outcome reached 24 points on the coma remission scale (Table 4) within the first 40 days of rehabilitation, none of the patients with less than 24 points on day 40 reached GOS 4 or 5. Also none of the patients with less than 10 points reached GOS more than 2.

Discussion

The first 6 weeks of early rehabilitation are extremely vulnerable for multiple complications, dominated by the brain and the respiratory system with short time need for invasive interventions. During the same time the patients have to experience those improvements, which are deciding the fate for a good recovery. So we have to provide an up-to-date monitoring for this time to prevent secondary damages which would affect especially those patients with a better rehabilitation potential. It is evident that short intervals

Table 4. *Coma Remission Scale*

Neurological-Neurosurgical Early Rehabilitation	**Coma Remission Scale (CRS)**	
Patient name:		
Date:		
Investigator (initials):		

1. **Arousability/attention** (to any stimulus)

Attention span for 1 minute or longer	5	
Attention remains on stimulus (longer than 5 sec)	4	
Turning towards a stimulus	3	
Spontaneous eye opening	2	
Eye opening in response to pain	1	
None	0	

2. **Motoric response** (minus 6 points from max. attainable sum if tetraplegic)

Spontaneous grasping (also from prone position)	6	
Localized movement in response to pain	5	
Body posture recognizable	4	
Unspecific movement in response to pain (vegetative or spastic pattern)	3	
Flexion in response to pain	2	
Extension in response to pain	1	
None	0	

3. **Response to acoustic stimuli** (e.g. clicker) (minus 3 points from max. attainable sum if deaf)

Recognizes a well-acquainted voice, music, etc.	3	
Eye opening, turning of head, perhaps smiling	2	
Vegetative reaction (startle)	1	
None	0	

4. **Response to visual stimuli** (minus 4 points from max. attainable sum if blind)

Recognizes pictures, persons, objects	4	
Follows pictures, persons, objects	3	
Fixates on pictures, persons, objects	2	
Occasional, random eye movements	1	
None	0	

between trauma and the beginning of early rehabilitation in a specialized facility will demand a full size intensive care management including all diagnostical and therapeutical resources. This includes methods for ICP/IVP measurement as well as invasive oxygen monitoring in brain tissue (Licox® system) [4], microdialysis [5, 6, 7] and Doppler sonography [8]. Of course raised intracranial pressure is a contraindication for rehabilitative therapies, but this does not exclude ICP measuring on an early rehabilitation unit if the patient is stable but still needs surveillance because of the short interval to his trauma. These methods do not only help us recording vital stress but also may indicate reactions of the comatose patient to coma stimulation therapy even though this will be subject of subsequent investigations.

The frequency and kind of neurosurgical secondary operations point out that this early phase of rehabilitation is an essential part of neurosurgical therapy to ensure continuity of treatment and to prevent transfers to other hospitals which will severely disturb reorganisation of the brain and reorientation of the patient returning from inconsciousness. One-hand-therapy assures surgery without loss of time in cases of emergency and also allows best possible timing of elective surgery, e.g. in cases of plastic reconstruction.

So 1/3 of all patients at the beginning of early rehabilitation still need invasive support for sufficient gas exchange, the usual hardware and experienced staff has to be provided. This includes invasive therapies such as endoscopy, which prevents numerous reintubations due to mucostasis, and knowledge of all current ventilation modalities. Although tracheostomy implies complications itself, we support early application in cases of neurogenic swallowing disorders because of a significant number of respiratory failures due to aspiration.

So the age pyramid changes to elderly people, we have to be aware of treating hemodynamic problems regularly. To measure medium arterial pressure, central venous pressure and peripheral oxygen saturation, should not be a problem today. A useful additional tool to control the benefits on the cerebral situation is the near infrared spectroscopy (NIRS, 9).

Metabolic changes are very common after head injuries, so routiners are controlling specific weight and sodium balance during the first weeks of the treatment.

Abdominal complications were not so common in our series, but they led to severe deterioration in single cases. We want to mention the case of an 80 year old patient, who died from sepsis after long lasting diarrhea, even without a definite diagnosis after necropsy.

Our results indicate that the mortality of those patients who survived up to the beginning of early rehabilitation is much lower than the mortality of the total due to the fact that most of the bad score patients dye within the first 10 days. The number of vegetative patients corresponds to the common reports [1, 3], allowing the assumption that persistent vegetative state (PVS) is still a problem of neurological medicine which cannot be solved by intensive rehabilitation alone. Of course it is disappointing that even under the best possible medical conditions the total number cannot be minimized. So the question arises for early prognostic parameters. Although experts agree that a temporary prognosis is allowed at the earliest after 6 months, we made the experience in our series that none of the patients with less than 10 points on the coma remission scale at day 40 of rehabilitation reached GOS > 2. Unaffected by this observation, we should look for statistically evaluated criteria of early prognosis. On the other hand, effective surgical, intensive care and early rehabilitative treatment can reach good outcomes in nearly half of the patients.

The results should encourage us to procede with the present way considering the fact that rehabilitation cannot reanimate functions we lost in the operation theatre or in the ICU. Since we are responsible for our complications in other diseases and operative procedures, we should insist to stay responsible for the complications during early rehabilitation of TBI patients.

References

1. Murray GD *et al* (1999) The European brain injury consortium survey of head injuries. Acta Neurochir (Wien) 141: 223–236
2. Gründe PO, Nordström CH (1998) Treatment of increased ICP in severe by head-injured patients. In: von Wild KRH, Nordström CH, Hernandez-Meyer F (eds) Pathophysiological principles and controversies in neurointensive care. W. Zuckschwerdt Verlag, München Bern Wien New York, pp 123–128
3. Bouillon B *et al* (1999) The incidence and outcome of severe brain trauma-design and first results of an epidemiological study in an urban area. Restorat Neurol Neurosc 14: 85–92
4. Meixensberger J *et al* (1993) Studies of pO₂ in normal and pathological human brain cortex. Acta Neurochir (Wien) [Suppl] 59: 58–63
5. Ungerstedt U *et al* (1998) Microdialysis monitoring of brain biochemistry during neurointensive care. In: von Wild KRH, Nordström CH, Hernandez-Meyer F (eds) Pathophysiological principles and controversies in neurointensive care. W. Zuckschwerdt Verlag, München Bern Wien New York, pp 83–90

6. Peerdemann SM *et al* (2000) Cerebral microdialysis as a new tool for neurometabolic monitoring. Int Care Med 26: 662–669
7. Landolt H *et al* (1996) Cerebral microdialysis as a diagnostic tool in acute brain injury. Eur J Anaesth 13: 269–278
8. Aaslid R *et al* (1982) Noninvasive transcranial Doppler ultrasound recording of flow velocity in basal cerebtal arteries. J Neurosurg 57: 769–774

9. Villringer A *et al* (1993) Near infrared spectroscopy (NIRS): a new tool to study hemodynamic changes during activation of brain function in human adults. Neurosci Lett 154: 101–104

Correspondence: Dr. med. Bernd Hoffmann, Clemenshospital Münster, Neurosurgical Department, Düesbergweg 124, 48153 Münster, Germany.

Acta Neurochir (2001) [Suppl] 79: 31–32

Early Functional Outcome in Isolated (TBI) and Combined Traumatic (CTBI) Brain Injury

E. Ortega-Suhrkamp

Asklepios Schloßberg-Klinik, Bad, Germany

Objectives

In the literature the longterm outcome of patients with combined traumatic brain injury is described considerably worse compared to patients with isolated traumatic brain injury only. Let me just point out Lehmann *et al.* [3], Gobiet [2], Broos *et al.* [1].

Keywords: Traumatic brain injury; intracerebral hemorrhage; early functional outcome.

Patients

Looking at some 448 accident victims, being discharged from our clinic between January, 1993 and December, 1998 we examined whether this statement could be confirmed already towards the end of early rehabilitation.

There were 270 patients with TBI, 76% male, 24% female, age 15 to 86 average age 42.9 years. 79% of the patients were treated primarily at a neurosurgical clinic, 21% of them at a general surgery. 178 patients suffered from CTBI, 80% male, 20% female, age 17–84, average age 35.2. Primary treatment was given at neurosurgery in 52%, at general surgery in 48%. According to acute care investigations available all patients were to be classified lower 8 on the Glasgow Coma Scale.

14.3% CTBI patients treated in general surgery only did not show any intracranial haemorrhage. 50% of these patients suffered from an isolated haemorrhage, whereas almost 90% of the patients treated primarily in neurosurgery showed a double or triple combination of haemorrhage. Among the group of isolated TBI only 4.7% of all patients treated in neurosurgery did not show intracranial haemorrhage, 29.7% showed an

isolated and 65% a double or triple haemorrhage. 40% of the patient group treated in general surgery showed an isolated, 60% a double or triple combination of haemorrhage.

Distribution of isolated haemorrhage in both patient groups: A subarachnoid haemorrhage was found in 6.3% of TBI and in 8.3% of CTBI. In both groups isolated concussion haemorrhage appeared most frequently.

Distribution of combined haemorrhage: In the CTBI group the combination of SAH and Concussion Haemorrhage predominates, whereas in the group of TBI the combination SAB, SDH and concussion haemorrhage prevail. 19% of TBI and 22% of CTBI suffered from an open head injury, 13% of TBI and 14% of combined TBI showed intracranial bleeding. In combined TBI there were the following attendant injuries: in 48% thoracic injuries, in 12% lung concussions, in 16% injuries of lungs and thorax, in 11% cardiac and abdominal injuries and in 80% 1 to 10 fractures of extremities, spine or pelvis.

Results

Based on discharge dates in 1998, early rehabilitation started on average after 33 days for patients with TBI, after 58 days for patients with CTBI. On the FIM-Scale CTBI reached 4 scores less, on the DRS 1 score less than the group of TBI.

In combined TBI early rehabilitation showed considerably longer duration with 102 days on average compared to TBI with 78 days.

During early rehabilitation CTBI showed more neurological complications in 8% compared to TBI, espe-

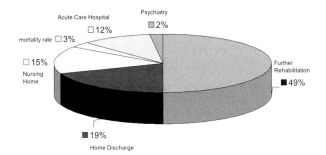

Fig. 1. Mode of discharge of patients with TBI

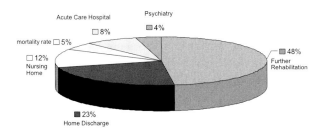

Fig. 2. Mode of discharge of patients with combined TBI

cially epilepsy, hydrocephalus and hygroma. Looking at the medical complications it is noticeable that all patients with CTBI developed medical problems which had to be treated: Nearly 50% of the patients developed more than 2 medical complications, specifically cardiac, pulmonary and/or gastrointestinal and urinary tract infections.

During early rehabilitation 3% of the patients with TBI died and 5% of the CTBI. The primary cause of death was of cardiac or of pulmonary origin.

Of those patients treated primarily in neurosurgery 78% of TBI and 69% of combined TBI improved in early rehabilitation, of those patients treated primarily in general surgery 71% of TBI and 75% of combined TBI improved.

Measured by the FIM-Scale the average scale addition in the group of TBI was 48.2, by the DRS 10.75 scores towards the group of combined TBI with 44.2, that is to say a scoring of 9.75 by the DRS.

The percentage of patients who were passed on to further rehabilitation was much the same in either group at 49/48% (Figs. 1 and 2).

Conclusion

Even though the acute care of patients with CTBI on average lasted 25 days longer, early rehabilitation 24 days longer and the mortality rate was 2% higher than in the comparing group of TBI, the outcome of those surviving was similar: Measured by the FIM-Scale there were 4 scores less, by the DRS 1 score less, putting TBI in favour. This result is also reflected in the mode of discharge: In either group just about half the patients were passed on to further rehabilitation. Therefore we conclude that we do not find confirmation of the worse longterm outcome of patients with combined TBI compared to patients with isolated TBI as is described in the literature in our patient group of 448 towards the end of early rehabilitation.

References

1. Broos PL, Stappaerts KH, Rommens PM (1998) Polytrauma in patients of 65 and over. Injury patterns and outcome. Int Surg 73(2): 119–122
2. Gobiet W (1995) Effect of mulitple trauma on rehabilitation of patients with craniocerebral injuries. Zentbl Chir 120(7): 544–550
3. Lehmann U, Steinbeck K, Gobiet W (1997) Prognose des polytraumatisierten Patienten mit schwerem Schädel-Hirntrauma während der Intensivphase. Langenbecks Arch Chir [Suppl] Kongressbd, S340–340

Correspondence: E. Ortega-Suhrkamp, Asklepios Schloßberg-Klinik, Frankfurter Straße 33, D-64732 Bad, Germany.

Acta Neurochir (2001) [Suppl] 79: 33–35

Neurological and Social Long-Term Outcome after Early Rehabilitation Following Traumatic Brain Injury. 5-Year Report on 240 TBI Patients

B. Hoffmann, C. Düwecke, and **K. R. H. von Wild**

Clemenshospital Münster, Neurosurgical Department, Academic Teaching Hospital of the Westfalian Wilhelms University Münster, Münster, Germany

Summary

The long term courses of patients after traumatic brain injury (TBI) are particularly influenced by the quality of neuropsychological rehabilitation and social reintegration. Though we do have data from different European countries about the success of surgery and intensive care, we don't know much about the long term courses, mirrored by the patients, their relatives and local physicians in their domestic environment. Supported by a pilot project of the government of Nordrhein – Westfalia we reviewed 252 patients with different grades of TBI, which were treated in our department from emergency to the end of early rehabilitation. At least 240 files could be completed, including observations up to 5 years after trauma (mean 26 months). 66% of the patients suffered from severe TBI according to the initial Glasgow Coma Scale (GCS), 23% showed moderate and 11% mild TBI. After discharge from early rehabilitation and during further treatment in rehabilitation hospitals patients with persistent vegetative state (PVS) did not show a significant benefit from therapy: Only 1 patient improved to GOS 3, fatal courses were observed in 3 patients, 11 patients remained unchanged. Patients with GOS 3 at the end of early rehabilitation on the other hand could improve in 51 cases to GOS 4 and 5. At the time of the actual investigation 32% of the patients reached GOS 5, 27% GOS 4. Unfavourable courses showed 21% (GOS 3), 5% (GOS 2) and 15% (GOS 1). Referred to the initial GCS only 16% of the severe, 27% of the moderate and 33% of the mild TBI could return to their former social activities and profession without any cuts. 145 of the total of surviving patients could return to their families, in the group of vegetative patients all except 1 patient were submitted for nursing homes. Only 58% of the patients practised any kind of outpatient rehabilitation, a specialized neuropsychological training has been restricted to 7% of the patients. So we observe a significant gap between a high impact clinical medicine on one side and a deficient outpatient treatment on the other. At least many patients are standing alone after discharge from rehabilitation hospitals, resulting in prolonged stationary treatment with extensive costs to minimize damage from this situation. Our consequence for a more efficient treatment is, that we substantially need better programs by local administrations, insurance companies and employers for better and earlier reintegration to avoid isolation and unnecessary invalidization, especially of those patients with the best medical prognosis.

Keywords: TBI; long term courses; social outcome; outpatient rehabilitation.

Introduction

Modern neurotraumatology does not only demand high standard operative neurosurgical treatment as well as sophisticated intensive care management for sufficient regulation of intracranial pressure, cerebral hemodynamics and metabolism but also implies the need for earliest beginning of rehabilitation to prevent the smallest traces of rehabilitation potential of the injured brain. Though we have detailed knowledge about many mechanisms that influence the early course and conditions of treatment after the onset of damage, we know much less about the late courses of surviving patients and the success or failure of reintegration into daily activities. So we wanted to analyze the social long – term outcome of a consecutive series of patients who were treated in our neurosurgical intensive care unit, followed by early rehabilitation in our neurosurgical early rehabilitation unit. This pilot project was made possible by the patronage of the government of Nordrhein – Westfalia, providing a specially designed unit for the treatment of at least 20 patients.

Patients and Methods

We reviewed 252 consecutive patients, who could be observed between 6 and 60 months (mean 26 months) after discharge from our department. Data were recruted from clinical findings, interview with the patient if possible as well as the relatives and the responsible physicians to acquire complete information about recent problems and the actual social situation. Complete files could be collected for 240 patients, so that the report concentrates on these patients. 165 (69%) of the patients were male, 75 (31%) were female. Age distribution showed a range between 14–87 years with a mean of 48 years. The age groups corresponded to other recent studies [2].

Results

The initial GCS score for the 240 patients was GCS 3–8 in 158 cases (66%), GCS 9–12 in 55 cases (23%) and GCS 13–15 in 27 patients (11%). Treatment in our early rehabilitation unit lasted 52 days as a mean. 160 patients were discharged to further rehabilitation in a rehabilitation hospital, 32 patients were discharged home for outpatient treatment, 25 patients went to nursing homes. 5 patients with severe psychiatric disorders were discharged to psychiatric hospitals, 7 patients with internal diseases to the medical department. Concerning the GOS outcome at the end of the treatment in our department as well as the final score at the time of recent examination we refer to Fig. 1. The patients' shift during the discharge from our unit and the time of follow up is demonstrated in Fig. 2. In the group of the vegetative patients only 1 improved to GOS 3, 3 patients died and 11 patients remained unchanged. Fifty-one patients with a GOS score of 3 at the end of early rehabilitation improved to GOS 4 and 5, 16 of them deteriorated and died. In GOS 4 28 patients improved and 9 patients deteriorated, in GOS 5 also 14 patients showed a worse late medical outcome. Retrospectively we observed that none of the patients with <20 (of 24) points in the coma remission scale at day 40 of treatment reached GOS 4 or 5 in the final,

also none of the patients with <10 CRS points at day 40 reached a GOS > 2. Of the surviving 204 patients 145 returned to their families, 36 still are living in nursing homes, 17 still stay in rehabilitation hospitals, 5 patients are in care of boarding schools and 1 is in prison. Depending on the initial GCS only 16% (26/158) of the GCS 3–8 patients returned to their former activities (school, apprenticeship, university, profession), 27% (15/55) in the GCS 9–12 group and 33% (9/27) with GCS 13–15. Depending on GOS at the end of early rehabilitation 15% (16/110) in the GOS 3 group showed normal activities, 24% (14/58) in GOS 4 and 43% (20/46) in GOS 5. In the long term course 52 patients retired, 10 patients are well rehabilitated but unemployed, 2 patients have to rely on social welfare, 2 patients are part time working and also 2 patients followed with the support of the job centre. Outpatient rehabilitation would have been necessary in 116 patients, but only 67 (58%) practised any kind of therapies. A specialized neuropsychological training was practised only in 7% of the patients.

Discussion

The results in the early stage, that means the results of surgical and intensive care therapy with early rehabilitation directly beginning after stabilization of intracranial pressure, are consistently mirroring the image of other recent studies [2, 5]. That implies that we reached a good international standard for this period in the patients' course. The low mortality is explained by the fact that we included only those patients surviving up to the beginning of early rehabilitation, because only this group is of interest in consideration of long term outcomes. On the other hand, the further course after early rehabilitation and the findings at the time of follow up enlighten surprisingly positive as well as disappointing facts. Early prognosis has always been difficult, especially in cases with suspected bad outcome. So it is important to see that the coma remission scale within the first 40 days of early rehabilitation reflects prediction of later long time outcome at least under selected conditions. This could be helpful to decide about continuation of hospital rehabilitation or outpatient treatment in long time nursing. The courses of vegetative patients remained serious, because only one of them developed active function even after a long period of early rehabilitation. The group of GOS 3 patients showed the best benefit of further rehabilitation so that intensive efforts are a "must do" in

Early rehab discharge			Long time results		
GOS	Number	%	GOS	Number	%
1	11	5	1	36	15
2	15	6	2	11	5
3	110	46	3	50	21
4	58	24	4	64	27
5	46	19	5	79	32

Fig. 1. GOS outcome score at the end of early rehabilitation (left) and at the time of follow up examination (right)

		GOS after long time rehabilitation					
		1	2	3	4	5	Total
GOS after early rehab	1	11					11
	2	3	11	1			15
	3	16		43	32	19	110
	4	4		5	21	28	58
	5	2		1	11	32	46
	Total	36	11	50	64	79	240

Fig. 2. Improvement or deterioration of patients' GOS outcome score after discharge from early rehabilitation

this entity. On the other hand, good function after early rehabilitation does not guarantee a good long-time outcome. Of course this is influenced by the fact that the changing age pyramid with growing numbers of elderly patients in our society enlarge the fact of co-morbidity in the further course. Happily most of the patients could return to their familiar homes after treatment, so that only 36 of the disabled patients needed help in nursing homes. So we can conclude that the recent medical efforts definitely achieve that most of the patients surviving brain injury have a distinct chance of quality and active function in daily life. Nevertheless there are significant problems in returning to former activities such as school, apprenticeship, university or profession. It does not surprise that success depends on initial GCS as well as the GOS outcome, the more it attracts attention that in 116 patients with need for ongoing outpatient therapies only 58% are practising one or more therapies with an alarming failure in neuropsychological support. Other authors [1, 3, 4] pointed out the background, needs and results of neuropsychological training for the improvement of cognitive functions as well as social behaviour so that it is not understandable that there is still such a difference to reality. In this context we interpret the large number of retired patients on the one side and the relatively small numbers of even good outcome patients who showed no handicap in social activities after brain injury on the other. Of course this problem does not only result from the lack of therapies but also from a lack of flexibility of the society including political conditions and the willingness of employers to make available adequate offers for the reintegration of disabled patients. So it is a fatal situation that the society obviously often prefers to pay for inability to work and unemployment instead of generating offers for reintegration respecting individual handicaps. So our conclusion under the aspects of long-time outcomes is that much more intense efforts must arise to use the success of medical treatment including intensive care medicine, early and long-time rehabilitation for a comparable success in social activities of the patients.

References

1. Barnes MP (1999) Rehabilitation after traumatic brain injury. Br Med Bull 55(4): 927–943
2. Bouillon B *et al* (1999) The incidence and outcome of severe brain trauma-design and first results of an epidemiological study in an urban area. Restorat Neurol Neurosc 14: 85–92
3. Carney N, Chesnut RM, Maynard H, Mann NC, Patterson P, Helfand M (1999) Effect of cognitive rehabilitation on outcomes for persons with traumatic brain injury. A systematic review. J Head Trauma Rehab 14(3): 277–307
4. Hellawell DJ, Taylor RT, Pentland B (1999) Cognitive and psychosocial outcome following moderate or severe traumatic brain injury. Brain Inj 13(7): 489–504
5. Murray GD *et al* (1999) The European brain injury consortium survey of head injuries. Acta Neurochir (Wien) 141: 223–236

Correspondence: Dr. med. Bernd Hoffmann, Clemenshospital Münster, Neurosurgical Department, Düesbergweg 124, 48153 Münster, Germany.

Acta Neurochir (2001) [Suppl] 79: 37–39
© Springer-Verlag 2001

Requirements of Team Effectiveness in Neurosurgical Rehabilitation

B. Kemper and **K. von Wild**

Clemenshospital, Department for Early Rehabilitation, Münster, Germany

Summary

The purpose of this article is to stress the importance of working with interdisciplinary teams in neurorehabilitation and describe requirements of team effectiveness. It is not sufficient to focus only on different impairments associated with brain injury and offer individuals a variety of therapy. The essential aspect in neurorehabilitation is the integration of disciplines and consistent goal setting to regard individual patient's needs. Interdisciplinary teams benefit from a leader qualified for neuroscience, neurorehabilitation, clinical neuropsychology and psychotherapy. A good structural organization of the team, notice of basic communication rules, understanding typical group dynamics and stressors of interdisciplinary teams, conflict management and a definite decision making increase productive interdisciplinary working and enable the team to continue to mature. Further empirical research is necessary to support the effectiveness of interdisciplinary teams as an important variable in the evaluation of rehabilitation outcome and quality control.

Keywords: Neurosurgical rehabilitation; team approach neuropsychology; interdisciplinary team.

Introduction

Cross-disciplinary developments in neuroscience have been exploding with great interest in understanding brain-behavior relationships, researching and treating patients with brain injury. Temporary or permanent loss of physical, motor, cognitive, behavioral and emotional functions and social problems after brain injury requires the integration of different disciplines (neuropsychologists, physicians, physical therapists, occupational therapists, social worker, speech therapists etc.) in the rehabilitation process.

The aim of our article is to outline the importance and requirements of "interdisciplinary team work" which can fulfill the high demands of modern neurorehabilitaton according to the ideas of holistic treatment.

Why have an Interdisciplinary Team?

The first and most important step in the process of neurological and neurosurgical rehabilitation is to clarify the neuropsychological diagnosis in order to plan the rehabilitation program. Beyond the etiology, the neuropsychological assessment must consider both impaired and preserved cerebral functions. It is necessary to understand the interdependency of primary and secondary impairments on neuropsychological functioning (e.g. How is a visual memory disturbance influenced by perceptual deficits?) Only information of different therapeutical disciplines regarding functional limitations, disabilities and social circumstances really allow a diagnosis and planning of a patient-specific rehabilitation.

The integration of behavioral observation, medical and familiar data and the influence or interaction with non-lesions variables is easier if the different disciplines work together and are integrated in the whole process of rehabilitation.

In this context it is important to stress the differences between multi- and interdisciplinary approaches. Of course, both offer a variety of therapeutical disciplines. But interdisciplinary teams are superior to multidisciplinary teams because better outcomes are accomplished by interactive efforts.

An interdisciplinary work increases the efficiency of rehabilitation. Efficiency means to avoid redundant, inconsistent and contradictory rehabilitation goals. Efficiency means to be flexible in structuring therapy schedules according the rehabilitation progress and the (psychological) needs of the patients. Efficiency means to work with families and benefit from the family's influence on the rehabilitation progress. Efficiency means that the staff learn from each other and share the burden of care, because working with brain dysfunctional patients produces affective reactions in both the patient's family and the rehabilitation staff.

In the light of a need for the integration among all the disciplines involved in the rehabilitation it is necessary to outline the requirements of interdisciplinary team work from a point of view of clinical neuropsychologist.

Requirements and Methods of Interdisciplinary Rehabilitation Work

The team needs a personality who is educated in interdisciplinary neuroscience and neurorehabilitation and benefits from a person, who is able to attend to the needs of the teams, patient, family and third-party payers. The leader must be alert to the role of group dynamics and stressors associated with interdisciplinary work. Problems often arise because the rehabilitation disciplines observe the same function or disturbances from different perspectives. Therefore the leader should avoid competition between the disciplines.

Because clinical neuropsychologists are qualified in neuroscience, in clinical neuropsychology, in psychotherapy and in communication they are predestinated for understanding brain-behavior abnormalities. Therefore interdisciplinary teams benefit from their knowledge and abilities to manage teams.

Besides the leader's qualification and personality, five other points should be mentioned which increase the efficiency of interdisciplinary team work:

Organization. A team needs a rehabilitation concept, regular and structured team meetings, support for further education in neurorehabilitation and clear sharings of tasks between the disciplines. It is not unusual that team members can become territorial rather than sharing the responsibilities of caring for patients.

Communication. Basic communication abilities include good listening, empathy, criticism, a respectful interaction with each other and abilities to accept different therapists' personalities.

Group Dynamics. It is necessary to foster an honest dialogue and to create a positive therapeutic milieu, in order to discuss controversially about the patient's disturbances and the content of rehabilitation. The staff needs structures which allow each member to apply his or her specific skills to help the patient. Every staff member should be included with equal rights independent of their disciplines. To be open for projections and own difficulties with patients and their families, a forum for review of patient-staff and staff-staff relations is absolutely necessary.

Conflict Management. Interdisciplinary team work inevitably arises conflicts. The team must be trained in problem solving in order to find out the reasons for difficulties. Team conflicts could be for instance explained by poor organization, problems in communication, neurobehavioral abnormalities of the patients etc.

Decision Making. A team wants and yet resists leadership. If the clinical director, who is usually responsible for the whole treatment of the patient, is really alert to the team's recommendations for the content and course of the rehabilitation, the staff will accept decisions. Hierarchical decision structures have negative effects on the therapeutic milieu.

These five points: organization, communication, group dynamics, conflict management and decision making are basic components which increase productive activity, creativity and motivation.

Conclusions

It is worthwhile to investigate time, energy and money in interdisciplinary team work, because these forms of cooperation really allow to identify the nature of brain-behavior abnormalities, to understand the consequences of the changes in the daily life of the individual and to contribute to effective and cost-efficient treatment of brain injury patients. Although the conclusion is accurate that the efficiency of interdisciplinary teams influence the rehabilitation outcome, empirical studies have neglected these aspects. The need for objective evaluation of neurorehabilitation outcome is crucial for establishing scientific credibility and quality control.

References

1. Fischer S, Trexler LE (1999) The CNR model of levels of functioning. Neuropsychol 10(2): 103–113

2. Prigatano GP (1999) Working with interdisciplinary rehabilitation teams. In: Prigatano GP (ed) Principles of neuropsychological rehabilitation. Oxford University Press, pp 228–243

3. Trexler LE, Helmke C (1996) Efficacy of holistic neuropsychological rehabilitation: Program characteristics and outcome research. In: Fries W (ed) Ambulante und teilstationäre Rehabilitation von Hirnverletzten. W. Zuckschwerdt Verlag, München, pp 25–40

Correspondance: Dr. phil Birgit Kemper, Clemenshospital, Academic Teaching Hospital of the University of Münster, Department for early Rehabilitation, Düesbergweg 124, 48153 Münster, Germany.

Acta Neurochir (2001) [Suppl] 79: 41–42

Merging Pathways: Music Therapy in Neurosurgical Rehabilitation

S. Gilbertson and **W. Ischebeck**

Klinik Holthausen, Hattingen, Germany

Summary

Relatively few departments of Music Therapy are found within neurosurgical rehabilitation clinics. In institutions where these departments exist, music therapy has become an integral part of multi-professional treatment and research activities (Gilbertson 1999).

The diverse intervention strategies in Music Therapy focus upon auditory, motor, visual, cognitive and affective processing which are all involved in receptive and expressive musical behaviour and which affect related non-musical behaviour. A clear differentiation is made between primary and adjunct therapy roles.

The related fields of neuromusicology, neuroanatomy, neuropsychology, music psychology and humanistic psychology are primary sources in the development of models of clinical application (Hodges 1996).

Our main interests are focussed on the following issues and areas of clinical application:

- The initialisation of contact with patients in vegetative status
- Communicative interaction with patients who can not (initially) use verbal communication (aphasic disorders)
- Temporal motor organisation with patients with sensomotor disorders
- Cognitive organisation and mnemonic framework with patients with neuropsychological functional disorders (concentration, memory, perception)
- Treatment of spatial perception disorders (neglect)
- Enhancing personal and social integration following individual isolation, social withdrawal

These topics will be discussed and highlighted with clinical examples.

Keywords: Neurorehabilitation music therapy.

Introduction

The development of music therapy specifically within neurosurgical rehabilitation began in Europe at the beginning of the 1990's. As the Klinik Holthausen, a clinic providing neurosurgical rehabilitation for 210 adults and 60 children opened in 1993, its Department of Music Therapy was one of the few of its type in existence within Europe. In the following years the Department expanded and now employs seven music therapists.

The Department provides both individual and group therapy in various modalities and is an integral part of a multi-professional team. Patients are referred by the ward doctors from all nine adult wards and both children's wards.

The Department is equipped to the highest standards and thus provides both the patients and therapists with the best possible environmental circumstances. Alongside providing therapy, the Department is also dedicated to supporting music therapy education through offering clinical placements for students.

Clinical Experiences and Conclusions

The term "Music Therapy" is a meta-category for a diverse range of therapeutic interventions, which are either augmentative, supportive or primary therapies, which are based on the medium of music (Hodges 1996).

The modalities of music therapy we offer include:

- Receptive Music Therapy
- Interactive Music Therapy
- Group Music Therapy
- Music-based motor rehabilitation

The following text presents an overview of the areas of clinical application and indications for these various forms of Music Therapy which have developed into core areas of clinical application during the past seven years (Gilbertson 1999):

The Initialisation of Contact with Patients in Vegetative Status

Aims at reaching the awareness of the patient which cannot be accessed through verbal communication. The music therapist improvises vocally to the breathing of the patient reflecting changes in intensity, tempo and dynamics. The patients' reactions observed in this phase are often minimal and subtle. A change in breathing, turning of the head in the direction of the therapist, the blinking of an eye, or the minute tapping of a finger can provide a platform for the development of simple, yet significant initial patterns of interaction.

Communicative Interaction with Patients with Aphasic Disorders

Offers the patient without expressive verbal ability a unique possibility to define and express their individual self in an expressive musical form. This is essential for the patients' development of personality and mood and thus the ability to re-enter into interpersonal relationships.

Temporal Motor Organisation with Patients with Sensomotor Disorders

Is applied for example, with patients with ataxia-the rhythmical structure of beating on a percussion instrument to rhythmical stimuli assists the co-ordination of muscle activity in arm movement which can significantly improve the fluidity and economy of movement patterns. Rhythmical stimuli are also used in the treatment of patients with hemiplegia during physiotherapy on the treadmill in the rehabilitation of ambulation.

Cognitive Organisation and Mnemonic Framework with Patients with Neuropsychological Functional Disorders

One example is a group therapy for patients with Organic Brain Syndrome being treated in our facul-tatively half-closed ward. During group improvisa-tions the patients are challenged with two main issues, firstly, the memory for musical fragments within the temporal organisation of improvised music undergoes extreme demands and secondly, they must learn to re-late and orient themselves to others within a non-directive group situation.

Treatment of Spatial Perception Disorders

Acoustic spatial awareness exercises are used to sig-nificantly increase spatial perception of contra-lateral hemispace in patients with Neglect syndrome.

Enhancing Personal and Social Reintegration Following Individual Isolation, Social Withdrawal

Many patients suffer not only from the loss of phys-iological and psychological function but also from the loss of their personal position in their ecological situa-tion.

The sharing of mutual aims, creation of personal objects (e.g. audio recordings) and a situation of close-ness with another person assists in reducing with-drawal and isolation commonly experienced follow-ing neurological illness. Furthermore, the patient can learn in a manner which is not solely based on coping mechanisms but based upon a striving towards per-sonal health.

References

1. Gilbertson S (1999) Music therapy in neurosurgical rehabilita-tion. In: Wigram T, De Backer J (eds) Clinical applications of music therapy in developmental disability, paediatrics and neu-rology. Jessica Kingsley Publishers, London, pp 224–245
2. Hodges D (1996) Neuromusical research. In: Hodges D (ed) Handbook of music psychology. IMR Press, San Antonio, pp 197–284

Correspondence: S. Gilbertson, Klinik Holthausen, Am Hagen 20, D-45527 Hattingen, Germany.

Acta Neurochir (2001) [Suppl] 79: 43–44

The Impact of Treatment on Survival Roles of a Person with a Traumatic Brain Injury

R. D. Voogt

Robert Voogt & Associates, Inc., Virginia Beach, VA

Summary

Over 250 survivors of brain injury were clinically evaluated and a long term care plan developed for each of them. 105 survivors were located and a follow-up questionnaire was administered at least two years later to the survivors and families to evaluate the predictions that were made regarding long-term needs.

The study looked at the impact on eight survival roles as defined by WHO and attempted to determine the effectiveness of services, correlating various treatment modalities and services with changes, adjustments, accommodations, achievements, and future goals. Results showed that there is a correlation between some non-traditional therapies (Recreational and Cognitive) and for individuals' future goals in physical independence, mobility, community reintergration and self care. These future goals were not significant for occupational and physical therapies. Also, a less significant correlatation was made between paid attendant care and level of outside activities.

Keywords: Head injury; treatment modalities; outcome.

A group of 272 individuals who had sustained traumatic brain injury were identified for use in this research project. Each of these individuals had been clinically evaluated as to their functional abilities and a long term care plan had been developed for each of them. In a follow-up study, 105 individuals were located that were willing to participate with their families in a questionnaire. This questionnaire was administered to them at least 2 years post the original clinical interview in order to evaluate whether the predictions made regarding their long term care needs were in fact, realized. In this study 73 males and 32 females participated. Twenty-six refused to participate, 6 individuals had died and 135 were never located. This questionnaire attempted to determine the effectiveness of various services correlating with various treatment modalities and services with changes, adjustments and accommodations, as well as achieve-

ments and the future goals that were envisioned by the survivors and their families. Of the 105 individuals that participated in this survey, 71% lived with their families, while 16% lived in a facility, 8% lived alone, and 5% lived with a roommate. Of the general population in the United States older than 25, only 5% live with their parents or an older relative.

In terms of employment, this research found that prior to their brain injuries, 54% of the participants had full time jobs, 9% had part time jobs, 31% were students, 1% were retired and 5% were unemployed. After the injury, 55% still remained unemployed, 18% considered themselves retired, 10% were students, 14% had part time jobs, 3% had full time jobs. It was interesting to note that only 1/3 of those who thought of themselves as retired, were older than 65. Some previous studies have indicated that the prognosis appears to be more optimistic where the injured individual has been engaged in post acute neuropsychological rehabilitation as it applies to employment. This current research found that receiving comprehensive rehabilitation did not significantly affect employment status. (P-Value $= 0.818$) What it did find, in fact, is that those who had received comprehensive rehabilitation were slightly less likely to be employed and more likely to consider themselves retired. In fact, of those who did receive this comprehensive neuropsychological rehabilitation, 15% were employed, 20% saw themselves as being retired, 48% remained unemployed and were not seeking employment. For those who did not receive this type of rehabilitation intervention, 21% were employed, 15% retired and 52% remained unemployed and were not seeking employment.

Another issue addressed was whether severity of injury affected current employment. Of the total of 105 individuals evaluated, 18 had sustained what was classified as mild injury. Forty-nine percent of this group was not looking for employment, 17% considered themselves retired, 17% were employed, 11% were students, and 6% were looking for employment. Of the 24 individuals who were considered to have a moderate injury, 55% were not looking for employment, 33% considered themselves retired, 8% were employed, 4% were students, and none were looking for employment within this grouping. The remainder of the group, with a population of 59, were considered to have sustained a severe brain injury. Forty-six percent were not looking, 14% considered themselves retired, 19% were employed, 14% were students, 7% were looking for employment.

The research also evaluated the effect that various therapies had on each of the individuals' outlook for the future. The various goals that were part of the questionnaire addressed the following areas: Physical independence and mobility; living situations; self care; community involvement; economic independence; occupation; education; interpersonal issues; and social. The results of the research show that the relationship between therapies and goals were not significant for individuals involved in occupational therapy ($P = 0.960$) and physical therapy ($P = 0.450$). However, there was a significant relationship ($P = 0.058$) between those who have been engaged in cognitive mediation and their future goals. It was also found that the individuals that had sustained traumatic brain injury were more likely than not to have goals if they had participated in recreational therapy. ($P = 0.067$) This is especially significant since traditional funding models, as well as the medical model, typically promote physical therapy and occupational therapy while cognitive remediation and recreational therapies have not been part of the main stream.

Finally, the research also found that individuals who had been involved in a structured rehabilitation program were more likely to be involved in outside activities. ($P = 0.004$) Of those who at the time of the survey were involved in a structured rehabilitation program, 78% reported participation in outside activities at least once per week. Of those who were not involved in a structured rehabilitation program, just 40% reported participation at that level. Of those who had never received any formal comprehensive rehabilitation, only 29% reported participation in outside activities at least once per week. Of interest is that of those who at the time of the survey received cognitive remediation, 82% reported participation in outside activities at least once per week.

In conclusion, it seems that more research tools and analyses are needed to measure what is effective at certain levels for long term improved outcomes. Functionally based rehabilitation will be necessary for the clients to achieve life and survivor goals. It is imperative that non-traditionally based therapies be evaluated for their usefulness within the rehabilitation models. Similarly, it is important to investigate why comprehensive rehabilitation does not make a significant impact on employment status. A further evaluation of our treatment models will be necessary so that improvements can be made to the delivery system.

References

1. Diller L, Ben-Yishay Yehuda (1987) Analyzing rehabilitation outcomes of persons with head injury. From rehabilitation outcomes; analysis and measure. Marcus J Fuhrer, Paul H Brookes Pub Co, Baltimore MD
2. Ezachi O, Ben Yishay Y, Kay T, Diller L (1991) Predicting employment in traumatic brain injury following neuropsychological rehabilitation. J Head Trauma Rehab 6: 71–84
3. Prigatano G, Klonoff PS, O'Brien KP et al (1995) Productivity after a neuropsychologically oriented milieu rehabilitation. J Head Trauma Rehab 9: 91–102
4. Sherer M, Madison CF, Hannay HJ (2000) A review of outcome after moderate and severe closed head injury with an introduction to life care planning. J Head Trauma Rehab 15(2): 767–782
5. Voogt R, Teasdale T, Patrick P, Carman J (1998) Reintegration into the family and the community following brain injury. Neuro-Rehab 11: 107–117

Correspondence: R. D. Voogt, Ph.D., C.R.C. 1055 Laskin Road, Suite 100 Virginia Beach, VA 23451.

Acta Neurochir (2001) [Suppl] 79: 45–47
© Springer-Verlag 2001

A Computerized Version of EBIS Evaluation Chart and its Opportunities in the Rehabilitation Program of TBI Patients

R. Avesani, Z. Cordioli, and **G. Salvi**

Dipartimento di Riabilitazione, Ospedale "S. Cuore – Don Calabria", Negrar-Verona, Italy

Summary

The need of rehabilitation programs for severely traumatic brain injured (TBI) patients is great and is growing, but these programs are long, costly and it would be very useful if we could demonstrate and quantify the benefits of our approaches.

We think that scarcity of literature in this field is a consequence of the well known and real difficulty in this kind of investigations (too many variability factors, groups of population not homogeneous, ethical problems for double blind studies and so on).

It is our opinion that EBIS Protocol could be a very useful instrument for the evaluation of rehabilitation programs benefits, provided that the protocol is used regularly for a long time after the acute phase and in many different TBI centres: in this way it would be possible to compare and to elaborate data concerning a large number of patients.

This instrument could also become an opportunity for a continuous and more coordinated collaboration between rehabilitation centres of different countries. We think that this target is realistic only if we dispose of a commonly accepted computerized version of EBIS Protocol with a data exchange via Internet.

Since 1996 we have been using a computerized version of the EBIS protocol for data archivation and follow up of TBI patients treated in our centre. The data bank concerns actually n. 341 TBI patients.

Objective of the present research is the presentation of a computerized version of EBIS protocol. This program is freely available and it could contribute to a more common use of this evaluation tool.

We thank particularly Prof. Truelle and Prof. Brooks who gave us the permission for the use of EBIS document.

Keywords: Rehabilitation; head injury; EBIS protocol.

Introduction

We think that actually the main priorities of research in the field of rehabilitation of the TBI are well summarized in the following statements:

"The focus of outcome studies that explores the benefits of trauma systems is mostly limited to issues of mortality and preventable deaths. Certainly, decreased mortality has a positive impact on society from both an economic and a social perspective. However there is a dearth of literature available on functional outcome. Such information could greatly expand the knowledge base regarding the impact of trauma systems. True reflection of benefit should be measured in terms of length of stay, cost, individual functional skills, independence and return to work and social activities" [1].

"Quelle est la qualité de vie de celui qui a été victime d'un traumatisme cranien grave?... Nos interventions leur ont réellement apporté quelque chose sur le plan qualitatif? Nous l'avons dit, l'optimisation de la qualité de vie du blessé et sa famille doivent rester l'objectif final du processus de rééducation et réadaptation et ces questions doivent rester la préoccupation constante des thérapeutes et des acteurs de la reinsertion tout au long de ce processus" [2].

EBIS protocol can become an important instrument for giving some responses to the above questions. With the present work we hope:

1. To show the easiness of use of the EBIS protocol in a computerized version, allowing the creation of a complete data bank, with the possibility of an immediate elaboration and correlation of all the items.
2. To contribute to a more expanded use of this instrument in all the European Centres dealing with TBI medical rehabilitation and social and vocational reintegration. A very quick information exchange could be easy by using Internet and every centre could potentially dispose of a common data bank.
3. It could then become easier to make a comparison of the evolution of similar groups of TBI patients, and a common research about the adequacy and

the efficacy of different (or similar) rehabilitation programs.

It is now useful to remind some of the EBIS protocol characteristics which are functional to the above mentioned aims:

a) EBIS protocol has been accepted in its actual form after repeated interdisciplinary and international meetings of TBI specialists and has been validated and utilized in a large TBI population in many European countries.
b) A large part of the protocol concerns social factors such as the reintegration and the quality of life of TBI patients. We think that these factors – in the evaluation of the long term outcome – are much more important than single specific scales. A global and "ecological" evaluation is highly significant in the complexity of the TBI disabilities and handicaps. R. L. Wood reminds that "the medical model is not suited to understanding disability and handicap because neither is exclusively a medical phenomenon and, indeed, the recent trend has been to emphasize social, cognitive and psychological factors as the essence of functional disability" [3].
c) It is required to fill in periodically the second part of EBIS protocol. In this way it becomes an instrument also for the rehabilitation program, making easier the patient follow up.

Material and Methods

EBIS protocol is composed of 175 items, divided into two main parts:

– the first part (52 items) concerns the initial phase: pretraumatic situation, types of injuries and symptoms in the acute phase
– the second part concerns post acute and long term outcomes considering:
  a) neuro motor, cognitive, emotional and behavioural fields
  b) familiar, social, scholastic and vocational reintegration

The software used in our Centre includes:

– *a first section* containing two programs with the exact original version of EBIS protocol and a data bank. For every patient, one can quickly see the entire evolution program.
– *a second section* which consists of a software program permitting every kind of statistical correlation of all items inserted in the data bank.

Since 1996, the EBIS protocol has been used for all TBI patients treated in our Intensive Rehabilitation Unit. The first part of the protocol is completed during the first 2 weeks after admission, the second part (follow up) at the end of the intensive rehabilitation phase. Next evaluations are done at 6 month or yearly intervals.

Results

This research concerns 341 TBI patients discharged from the hospital in the years 1996–2000. The percentage of "lost" patients is 25% at second follow-up and 40% at third follow-up.

We are now reporting only a few examples of data elaboration, just to show how the software program works.

The data concern: categories of TBI population (Table 1), types of accident (Table 2) and correlation between gravity of initial injury (Table 3) and functional outcomes (Table 4) (referring only the Glasgow Outcome Scale).

Table 1. *Activity Before Accident (Item n. 10)*

Full-time job	53.3%
Part-time job	4.0%
Retired	13.4%
Unemployed	5.5%
Housework	4.4%
Child	0.5%
Student	13.6%
Others	5.3%

Table 2. *Type of Accident (Item n. 24)*

Driver	19.7%
Passenger	11.9%
Pedestrian	5.5%
Motor-cycle	33.1%
Bicycle	6.4%
Sport accident	2.0%
Domestic	10.1%
Assault	0.5%
Others	10.8%

Table 3. *GOS (Item n. 175) at 3, 6, 12 Months after Injury*

	1° follow up	2° follow up	3° follow up
GOS 1	34%	56%	61%
GOS 2	33%	21%	17%
GOS 3	31%	21%	20%
GOS 4	2%	2%	2%

Table 4. *PTA (Item 29) and GOS Correlation: 12 Months after Injury*

	PTA 8–28 days	PTA 28–60 days	PTA > 60 days
GOS 1	100%	56%	34%
GOS 2	0%	23%	33%
GOS 3	0%	21%	31%
GOS 4	0%	0%	2%

Job reintegration (12 months after injury): 37% (from a total of 173 persons employed before injury).

Conclusions

EBIS Protocol in its computerized version is an easily used evaluation instrument combining the quality of the original protocol and the versatility of a computerized program. The program is freely available for all interested centres.

It is the opinion of the AA that a coordinated use of this system in different European TBI Centres could permit:

1. a periodical comparison via Internet of recorded data.
2. a stimulus to research in the rehabilitation field, because of the large number of available data.
3. a reciprocal comparison of different rehabilitation programs, of the evolution over time and of final functional outcomes of homogeneous groups of TBI patients.
4. new opportunities for a more frequent exchange of views between specialists of different Rehabilitation Centres.

References

1. Cohadon F *et al* (1998) Les traumatisés craniens, de l'accident à la reinsertion, Arnette, Paris, p 315
2. Mackay LE *et al* (1997) Maximizing brain injury recovery: integrating critical care and early rehabilitation. Aspen publ., p 22
3. Wood RL, Eames P (1989) Models of brain injury rehabilitation. Chapman and Hall Ltd, pp 96–97

Correspondence: R. Avesani, Dipartimento di Riabilitazione, Ospedale "S. Cuore – Don Calabria", Negrar-Verona, Italy.

Acta Neurochir (2001) [Suppl] 79: 49–51

Satisfaction of Life and Late Psycho-Social Outcome after Severe Brain Injury: A Nine-Year Follow-up Study in Aquitaine

J. M. Mazaux[2], **P. Croze**[1], **B. Quintard**[1], **L. Rouxel**[2], **P. A. Joseph**[2], **E. Richer**[3], **X. Debelleix**[3], and **M. Barat**[2]

[1] Laboratoire de Psychologie EA 526 et Groupe Handicap et Cognition EA 487, Université de Bordeaux 2, France
[2] Service MPR, Hôpital Pellegrin, CHU de Bordeaux, Bordeaux, France
[3] Réseau UEROS Aquitaine, Centre Château Rauzé, Centre de la Tour de Gassies, Bruges, France

Summary

In view of assessing their late outcome and satisfaction of life, 79 out of 158 severe traumatic brain injury (STBI) patients who received inpatient rehabilitation in Aquitaine in 1993 were followed by phone interview. Results showed that 9 years on average after their injury, 65 to 85% of these patients were independent for daily living, whereas 35 to 55% only were independent in social life. Most of the patients were satisfied with their autonomy (67%), family life (66%) and financial status (41%), but they were dissatisfied with leisures (36%), vocational adjustment (28%) and sexual life (32%). Satisfaction of life was mostly related to age, gender, physical autonomy, need of help because of cognitive impairment and functional outcome as assessed by the Glasgow Outcome Scale.

Severe traumatic brain injury (STBI) stands in industrialised countries as a major Public Health problem and a dreadful human drama for the patients, their families and the community [2]. A great number of STBI patients survive with severe disability, most of them being young adults. The most severely impaired may live only with their parents or in high-cost nursing homes. From a psychological point of view, STBI causes a total and sudden breakdown of the mental states, personality and conditions of life. Life plans and projects are definitively disrupted, satisfaction of life is deeply changed.

Rehabilitation aims at improving functional outcome of persons with STBI, and at improving their overall quality of life. Planning for rehabilitation and re-entry into community of STBI patients need to be provided with precise data on their late outcome and disability level. Despite that the concepts of quality and satisfaction of life are difficult to define and moreover to assess, these are also major factors to take into account.

The aims of the present study were to assess the late psycho-social outcome of patients hospitalized in Aquitaine for rehabilitation of a STBI 7 to 10 years after their injury, and to ask for their satisfaction of life and subjective feeling of quality of life.

Keywords: Traumatic brain injury; psycho-social outcome rehabilitation.

Method

Patients

Fourteen of the 17 hospitals and rehabilitation centers admitting STBI patients for rehabilitation in Aquitaine accepted to participate in the study. Patients were enrolled if they had been hospitalized in one of these units during the year 1993, and if they suffered a STBI as defined by a Glasgow coma scale score of eight or below during the first 24 hours out of neuro-sedation, or a score over 8 with secondary worsening and neursurgical intervention. One-hundred fifty-eight patients fulfilling these criterias were included. We could find again and contact only 105 of them. Ten were dead, 16 refused to answer or did not provide complete data. Finally, 79 qestionnaires were available.

Method

Patients were asked for by phone interview. The Glasgow Outcome Scale (GOS) was used to assess overall outcome. Twenty-five items of the French version of the European EBIS Document [1] were completed from interview to assess autonomy in daily living, behavior and disability level. A 9-item Satisfaction of Life Scale [3] and open questions were used to assess subjective feelings of quality of life, satisfaction with treatment and psycho-social issues. Data were collected and treated with softwares SPSS 7.5 and Statbox.

Results

Patients in sample were 69 men (71%) and 20 women (29%). Mean age was 40,5 years. The mean coma duration was 29 days, and mean time since injury 9,24 years. Twenty-two patients had a good recovery (GOS 1: 24.7%), 38 a moderate disability (GOS 2: 42.7%), 24 a severe disability (GOS 3: 27), and 5 were in a

Table 1. *EBIS Document: Autonomy Rates in Daily Living and in Social Life*

Activity	Percentage
Eating	84,81
Bladder and bowel control	81,7
Grooming	65,8
Dressing	63,3
Standing	74,7
Moving inside the home	70,9
Moving outside	64,6
Shopping	53,2
Writing letters	51,9
Using public transports	61
Driving a car	37
Performing administrative tasks	35,9

Table 2. *Subjective Assessment of Satisfaction of Life and Most Important Domains for Quality of Life in Sample*

Satisfaction of life domain	Satisfaction	SWC	Most important
Life as a whole	35	73	–
Autonomy	67	94	19
Leisure	36	56	1,6
Work status	28	59	27
Financial status	41	47	4,8
Sexual life	32	67	3,2
Marital life	52	77	14,3
Family life	66	82	22,2
Relationships with friends	55	59	7,9

SWC Swedish controls.

vegetative state (GOS 4: 5.6%). Ten patients were living in nursing homes.

Autonomy rates in daily living were assessed by the EBIS Document (Table 1). As a whole, 65 to 80% of patients were independent for personal and domestic activities such as eating, dressing, grooming or moving inside the home, whereas 35 to 55% only were independent in social life. For instance, only half the patients were able to do shopping or to write letters, and one third were able to drive a car or to perform administrative tasks. Fourteen percent of patients needed help in daily living for physical reasons, other 14% for mental reasons, and 44.8% needed legal assistance in social life.

With regard to work status, 19% of patients returned to a full-time work at the date of the study, 7% were working part-time, and 9,5% had sheltered employment. Nine percent were still students and 5,5% were unable to work or to study any more. Thirty-six percent of patients had the same leisure than before the injury, 30% developed new ones (mostly sedentary activities such as reading or watching TV) and 34% had no leisure any more. Family members' burden was assessed important to unbearable in nearly 44% of cases.

Satisfaction of life was assessed by the Fugl-Meyer's scale in comparison with Swedish health controls of similar age and education (Table 2). Thirty-five percent of patients only were satisfied with their life as a whole. Patients were mostly satisfied with their family life and physical autonomy, and were mostly dissatisfied with their work status (28%) with their leisure (36%) and with their sexual life (32%). They said to be satisfied with treatment and rehabilitation (88.8%).

We are unable to provide in this short-form paper

further data, including comparisons with French controls, results of two principal component analyses and results of multiple linear regressions used for assessing the influence of demographic data, disability level and global outcome on satisfaction of life. They will be published later.

Discussion

Consistently with previous studies [6, 8] we observed a clear dissociation between basic autonomy for daily living, and participation in social life with high cognitive and behavioral demand. So cognitive rehabilitation and social education are prioritary to develop in order to improve the late outcome of STBI patients. Previous works outlined the importance of physical autonomy, psychological well-being and return to work as critical factors of quality of life in STBI patients [4, 5, 9]. In our study most of the patients were satisfied with their autonomy, family life and financial status, but they were dissatisfied with leisures, vocational adjustment and sexual life. This reminds us of Prigatano's famous words «work, love and play» [7]. And these should be prioritary goals to target when planning rehabilitation in view of improving satisfaction of life after traumatic brain injury.

References

1. Brooks N, Truelle JL *et al* (1995) Document Européen d'évaluation des traumatisés crâniens. EBIS, Bruxelles
2. Cohadon F, Castel JP, Richer E, Loiseau H (1998) Les traumatisés crâniens: de l'accident à la réinsertion. Arnette, Paris
3. Fugl-Meyer A, Branholm I, Fugl-Meyer K (1991) Happiness and domain – specific life satisfaction in adult northern Swedes. Clin Rehab 5: 25–33

4. Joseph PA, Le Gall D, Aubin G, Forgeau M, Truelle JL (1995) Evaluation de la qualité de vie par les traumatisés crâniens et par leur entourage. In: Hérisson C, Simon L (eds) Evaluation de la qualité de vie. Masson, Paris, pp 189–194
5. Klonoff P, Snow W, Costa L (1986) Quality of life in patients 2 to 4 years after closed head injury. Neurosurgery 19(5): 735–743
6. Ponsford J, Olver J, Curran C (1995) A profile of outcome: 2-years after traumatic brain injury. Brain Inj 9: 1–10
7. Prigatano G (1989) Work, love and play after brain injury. Bull Menninger Clin 53(5): 414–431
8. Tate R, Lulham J, Broe G, Strettles B, Pfaff A (1989) Psychosocial outcome for the survivors of severe blunt head injury: the results from a consecutive series of 100 patients. J Neurol Neurosurg Psychiatry 52: 1128–1134
9. Webb C, Wrigley M, Yoels W, Fine P (1995) Explaining quality of life for persons with traumatic brain injury 2 years after injury. Arch Phys Med Rehab 76: 1113–1119

Correspondence: J. M. Mazaux, Service MPR, Hôpital Pellegrin, CHU de Bordeaux, Bordeaux, France.

Acta Neurochir (2001) [Suppl] 79: 53–57

Clinical Efficacy of Stimulation Programs Aimed at Reversing Coma or Vegetative State (VS) Following Traumatic Brain Injury

M. Vanier[1,2], **J. Lamoureux**[1], **E. Dutil**[1,2], and **S. Houde**[2]

[1] Université de Montréal, Montréal, Québec, Canada
[2] Institut de réadaptation de Montréal, Montréal, Québec, Canada

Introduction

«Therapy aimed at reversing the persistent vegetative state has not been successful» [2]. This is one conclusion of the report of the Multi-Society Task Force on PVS, which examined the medical aspects of the persistent vegetative state (PVS). Although controversial, stimulation interventions for patients in PVS after an acute brain injury are an element of clinical practice in many countries, both for ethical and for scientific reasons, until enough knowledge is accumulated on this clinical entity. Present methods of treatment and their scientific rationale, expected levels of improvement in consciousness due to treatments and research methodologies for outcome studies appropriate for this rare and very variable clinical condition are not well known in the scientific literature. As Cope [4] mentioned in his analysis of the effectiveness of traumatic brain injury (TBI) rehabilitation in general, there is a large number of «outcome studies» of TBI rehabilitation but the vast majority of these do little to help resolve the issue of efficacy, as they fail to address issues of pre- and post-treatment function, spontaneous recovery, definition of severity of injury and other methodological problems. This is particularly true for the stimulation programs for patients in PVS. Analysis of existing scientific publications on the efficacy of these interventions is required to disentangle the present situation in which clinicians feel the necessity to do something for their patients but are restrained by conflicting opinions in the literature and the resulting disinterest of researchers. A non-wanted effect of the absence of critical studies is a drastic change in hospital policy, resulting in the interruption of stimulation interventions without and before a demonstration of their efficacy/inefficacy. To bring additional light to this complex clinical situation, this paper critically reviews scientific publications addressing the clinical efficacy of stimulation interventions for patients in coma or in vegetative state.

Keywords: Rehabilitation; traumatic brain injury stimulation programmes.

Methods

The reviewed studies were selected on the basis of the following criteria: (1) Study groups consisting mainly of patients considered in coma or in vegetative state; if minimally responsive (MR) patients were included, they had to be studied separately. (2) A description of the pre/post program *level of consciousness* of the patients. (3) A description of the stimulation program. (4) An evaluation of the program in terms of its clinical efficacy. The search was done through medical databases (Medline, Psychinfo: 1966–1998) and publications cited in the reference list of relevant articles.

To determine the efficacy of a treatment, researchers rely on empirical data. The reliability of the conclusions of empirical research is influenced by [25]: (1) *construct validity*, which corresponds to the extent to which the theoretical constructs have been successfully operationalized within the study; the construct validity of a study emphasises the importance of appropriately measuring the dependent and independent variables of interest; (2) *external validity*, which corresponds to the extent to which the detected outcomes are generalised to other subjects or situations; (3) *internal validity*, which corresponds to the extent to which the detected outcomes are caused by the controlled variables defined in the study; the internal validity explores the possibility of rival explanations into treatment effects; (4) *statistical validity*, which is defined as the sensitivity or the power of the design to detect outcome effects; the statistical validity explores the implications of sampling variations in the explanation of the relations observed between the treatment and the outcome. Each of these four aspects of the validity was examined in the selected studies.

Results and Discussion

A total of 563 published studies were identified that considered one or the other of the criteria specified. Three types of programs were identified: neurostimulation, psychostimulant pharmacotherapy and sensory stimulation. Among these, 36 articles included both a description and an evaluation of a stimulation program, 16 of which included a pre/post-program evaluation; these last studies [5, 6, 8, 9, 12, 14–16, 18–20, 22, 23, 26–28] were selected for analysis and presented in this paper. The complete list of studies is available from the first author (MV) upon request.

Construct Validity: Level of Consciousness

Most authors use a qualitative description of the behaviour of the patient as well as the Glasgow coma scale (GCS) [24] to determine the level of consciousness. When other instruments are used, they belong to the categories of scales measuring changes from coma to the end of post-traumatic amnesia (Sensory Stimulation Assessment Measure [21], Western Sensory Stimulation Profile [3], *Fiche Synthèse* [22]) or changes from coma to social independence [17]. Analysis of these instruments, following Horn *et al.* [11], indicates that, among these scales, only the GCS uses the level of consciousness as the measured variable. The other scales measure variables such as «response to stimulation» (with a specification that the instrument does not measure consciousness), «cognitive organisation», «many behavioural variables». In some cases, the concept measured is not specified. The GCS is a valid instrument but it is relatively insensitive to change from coma to VS to consciousness. Other instruments, like the Rancho and the FS, include non-mutually exclusive large categories that make impossible the measure of the level of consciousness. Instruments like the SSAM and the WSSP are too recent and have not been fully validated at the time of the studies. Both the descriptions and the scales, published between 1974 and 1994 (starting in 1969, for the descriptions) reflect various changes in the definition of altered states of consciousness during this period. For that reason, results of outcome studies must be examined with a special attention to the concepts measured by these scales and descriptions. On table 1, are presented examples of definitions of concepts in three different studies. As is shown, labels are used for «coma» and «comatose state» without conceptual definitions. Also the operational definition, or measure, of the variables «coma», «comatose» and «vegetative state» are not mutually exclusive: what is considered a «vegetative state» in Wood *et al.*'s study [28] (GCS score of 9 or 10) is included in the category «moderate coma» in Kater's study [15] (GCS: 7–10) and is included in the category «comatose» in Jones *et al.*'s study [13] (Level II on the Rancho). From the inconsistencies in the operationalisation of the level of consciousness, it becomes impossible to compare these programs in terms of efficacy.

Construct and External Validity: Stimulation Program

Neurostimulation is aimed at stimulating the nervous structures directly or indirectly involved in the arousal system and at stimulating the metabolic system (cerebral blood flow, glucose metabolism and oxygen consumption). Three studies [9, 14, 18] report pre/post-program results. Two types of effect of neurostimulation are invoked on the basis of experimental results: a non-specific cortical activation, manifested in behaviour by an arousal response, and a more global effect, described as improvement in clinical status. No study provides sufficient information on the program used to render it reproducible for further studies.

Psychostimulant pharmacological treatment consists in the administration of medication aiming at promoting arousal and consciousness. Five studies [5, 6,

Table 1. *Conceptual and Operational Definitions of Coma, Comatose State and Vegetative State in Three Studies*

	Coma (Kater [15])	Comatose (Jones [13])	Vegetative state (wood [28])
Conceptual definition	none presented	none presented	sleep/wake cycles and other characteristics indicative of VS
Operational definition	coma GCS deep: 3–6 moderate: 7–10 light: 11–14	level II on the Rancho ("generalized, nonpurposeful responses to a variety of sensory stimuli")	GCS: 9 or 10 level II or III on the Rancho

16, 26, 27] report pre/post-program results. The effects of the medications invoked in the studies reviewed are (1) improvement in patients with an apallic syndrome and in patients in *prolonged coma* treated with L-Dopa, (2) improvement of the level of activity, the attention span and sleep and eating habits in hyperactive children treated with Sinemet and (3) a marked increase in cerebral glucose consumption and oxydation in conscious brain lesioned patients. Four studies provide very incomplete information on program duration.

Sensory stimulation programs consist in the presentation of stimuli in one or many sensory modalities to promote return of consciousness. There are multimodal and unimodal sensory stimulation programs and one program advocating the regulation of the sensory environment. Nine studies [8, 12, 15, 19, 20, 22, 23] report pre/post-program results. In these, theoretical arguments are proposed but only two types of effects of sensory stimulation based on experimental results are invoked: stimulation in conscious children with developmental retardation diminishes this retardation and increases psychosocial performance; physiological changes, such as an increase in size and weight of the brain, occur when animals are in a stimulating environment. The experiments referred to do not share the same variables as those used in the clinical studies on unconscious patients. None of the studies provide enough information to allow replication.

Internal Validity: Study Designs

Table 2 illustrates the distribution of study designs according to the type of stimulation used. Few of the 16 studies reviewed had a solid enough design to eliminate rivalling explanation in the variation of the outcome variable.

Two randomised controlled trials were done but the samples were small (n = 14 and n = 19), and the ran-domisation process was lost on such small samples; the compared groups were not comparable even with the randomisation. There were two non-randomised trials with matched groups. Both of them were done with historical controls. Due to the rapid evolution of the field and the lack of consistency in the definition of the level of consciousness between studies, historical controls may not be comparable to experimental patients. Four of the 16 studies used a non-randomised, non-matched, controlled design. This design does not allow comparison of treatment effect between groups. The most common design was the single group design (seven) which does not give evidence of the efficacy of treatment. The fact that researchers use this design emphasizes the issue of small sample size. Six out of the seven studies using a single group design had less than 15 subjects included. Separating those subjects into subgroups would have created a problem of statistical validity.

Only one of the 16 studies used a single case (chronological series) design. If researchers use this design more often in the future, and effectively measure the program effect on the level of consciousness of individuals, it will become possible to perform meta-analyses to generalise program effect on the level of consciousness.

External and Statistical Validity: Sample Selection and Statistical Analyses

Six studies (two on neurostimulation, two on pharmacological stimulation and two on sensory stimulation) report selection criteria for their sample. For the other ten studies, we do not know to what population the findings can be generalised. Therefore those ten studies lack external validity.

The sampling method is an important statistical criterion. The only single-case study reports a random sampling of the measures which is appropriate for that

Table 2.

	Neurostimulation	Pharmacological treatment	Sensory stimulation
Randomised controlled trial (RCT)	1	0	1
Non-randomised matched controlled trial	0	0	2
Non-randomised controlled trial	0	1	3
Single group	2	4	1
Single case	0	0	1

design. In this type of study, if a random sampling of the measures is imperative, so is the description of the subject(s) assessed. A single-case experiment is most useful if its results can eventually be combined with the results of other single-case experiments. For this to be possible, the subjects must be described extensively in order to eventually combine subjects that have common characteristics. Unfortunately, the single-case experiment reviewed did not describe in details the subjects studied.

In quantitative evaluative research, statistical testing is the tool used to determine treatment efficacy. Eleven out of the 16 studies use some kind of measure (GCS, Rancho, GOS, etc) to quantify the level of consciousness but only five report statistical analyses to determine if the program had an effect on the outcome; however, none of these five studies justified the sample size used.

Statistical analyses are tools to prove that the changes observed in the level of consciousness are due to treatment effect and not to chance. This is true only if a random process is introduced at one point in the study (random selection of subjects, randomisation of the selected subjects between groups, random sampling of measures, etc.). Since only three studies use a random process (two randomised-controlled trials and one single-case study), it follows that statistical analyses were methodologically appropriate only in those instances.

Conclusion

Although there exists an important number of publications on interventions aiming at reversing the unconscious state resulting from acute brain injury, a very small proportion of them addresses the question of efficacy of these interventions. Sixteen scientific publications on efficacy have been identified and analyzed in terms of the four standard aspects of validity (construct, external, internal and statistical validity).

There is no consensus on how to measure the dependent variable, the level of consciousness. In addition, the theoretical bases of the stimulation programs are surprisingly underdeveloped in many studies. In further studies the researcher should give considerably more attention to construct validity. Very few studies provide sufficient information on the program used to render it reproducible for further studies. Again, few of the publications reviewed had a solid enough design to eliminate rivalling explanation in the variation of

the outcome variable. Because few studies report selection criteria for their sample, we do not know to what population the findings can be generalised. Only five studies report statistical analyses to determine if the program had an effect on the outcome, but none of them justified the sample size used.

Considering the wide heterogeneity of the population of patients in coma or in vegetative state [1, 7] and the small number of patients available for study at any one time, two approaches can be suggested in future research for the determination of stimulation program effect. The first approach is a multicenter randomised controlled trial. Multicenter studies increase the number of available subjects but have the disadvantage of very high costs; their planning requires intense teamwork and is time-consuming. This approach is therefore not available to every clinician working in the field, for whom a second approach can be suggested, the single-case experiment. Single-case experiments are easy to plan, cost very little and, when the researcher has a certain number of experiments, can be analysed together to provide some sort of generalisability to the population of interest [10]. Adequate planning can help attain statistical validity within the frame of single-case experiments. First, the clinician should identify the dependent variable and its measure. He should then select the appropriate statistical test to evaluate treatment efficacy, determine the level of statistical error and the desired power of the test and calculate the sample size (in this case the number of measures) needed to identify clinically significant treatment efficacy.

This research has been funded by the *Société de l'assurance automobile du Québec* and the *Fonds de recherche en santé du Québec* (Grant # 941298).

References

1. Andrews FM, Klem L, Davidson TN, O'Malley PM, Rodgers WL (1981) A guide for selecting statistical techniques for analyzing social science data, 2nd edn. University of Michigan, Ann Arbor, 70 pages
2. Anonymous (1994) Medical aspects of the persistent vegetative state (2). The Multi-Society Task Force on PVS. New Engl J Med 330(21): 1572–1579
3. Ansell BJ, Keenan JE (1989) The Western Neuro-Sensory Stimulation Profile. A tool for assessing slow-to-recover head injured patients. Arch Physic Med Rehab 70: 104–108
4. Cope DN (1995) The effectiveness of traumatic brain injury rehabilitation: a review. Brain Inj 9(7): 649–670
5. Dalle Ore G, Bricolo A, Alexandre A (1980) The influence of the administration of pyritinol on the clinical course of traumatic coma. J Neurosurg Sci 24(1): 1–8
6. Di Rocco C, Maira G, Meglio M, Rossi GF (1974) L-Dopa

treatment of comatose states due to cerebral lesions. Preliminary findings. J Neurosurg Sci 18(3): 169–176

7. Giacino JT (1996) Sensory stimulation: theoretical perspectives and the evidence for effectiveness. NeuroRehab 6: 69–78

8. Hall ME, MacDonald S, Young GC (1992) The effectiveness of directed multisensory stimulation versus non-directed stimulation in comatose CHI patients: pilot study of a single subject design. Brain Inj 6(5): 435–445

9. Hassler R, Ore GD, Dieckmann G, Bricolo A, Dolce G (1969) Behavioural and EEG arousal induced by stimulation of unspecific projection systems in a patient with post-traumatic apallic syndrome. Electroencephalography Clin Neurophysiol 27(3): 306–310

10. Hershberger SL, Wallace DD, Green SB, Marquis JG (1999) Meta-analysis of single-case designs. Statistical strategies for small sample research. In: Hoyle RH (ed) Thousand Oaks, Sage, pp 107–132

11. Horn S, Shiel A, McLellan L, Campbell M, Watson M, Wilson B (1993) A review of behavioural assessment scales for monitoring recovery in and after coma with pilot data on a new scale of visual awareness. Neuropsychol Rehab 3(2): 121–137

12. Johnson DA, Roethig Johnston K, Richards D (1993) Biochemical and physiological parameters of recovery in acute severe head injury: responses to multisensory stimulation. Brain Inj 7(6): 491–499

13. Jones R, Hux K, Morton-Anderson KA, Knepper L (1994) Auditory stimulation effect on a comatose survivor of traumatic brain injury. Arch Physic Med Rehab 75(2): 164–171

14. Katayama Y, Tsubokawa T, Yamamoto T, Hirayama T, Miyazaki S, Koyama S (1991) Characterization and modification of brain activity with deep brain stimulation in patients in a persistent vegetative state: pain-related late positive component of cerebral evoked potential. Pacing Clin Electrophysiol 14(1): 116–121

15. Kater KM (1989) Response of head-injured patients to sensory stimulation. West J Nursing Res 11(1): 20–33

16. Lal S, Merbtiz CP, Grip JC (1988) Modification of function in head-injured patients with Sinemet. Brain Inj 2(3): 225–233

17. Malkmus D (1980) Cognitive assessment and goal setting. In

Rehabilitation of the head injured adult: conprehensive management. Professional staff association of Rancho Los Amigos Hospital Inc, pp 1–11

18. McLardy T, Mark V, Scoville W, Sweet W (1969) Pathology in diffuse projection system preventing brainstem-electrode arousal from traumatic coma. Confinia Neurol 31(4): 219–225

19. Mitchell S, Bradley VA, Welch JL, Britton PG (1990) Coma arousal procedure: a therapeutic intervention in the treatment of head injury. Brain Inj 4(3): 273–279

20. Pierce JP, Lyle DM, Quine S, Evans NJ, Morris J, Fearnside MR (1990) The effectiveness of coma arousal intervention. Brain Inj 4(2): 191–197

21. Rader MA, Alston JB, Ellis DW (1989) Sensory stimulation of severely brain-injured patients. Brain Inj 3(2): 141–147

22. Rapin PA, Richer E (1994) Intérêt d'une prise en compte de la dimension relationnelle lors de la prise en charge en phase d'éveil de coma. Journal de réadaptation médicale 14(3): 123–130

23. Sisson R (1990) Effects of auditory stimuli on comatose patients with head injury. Heart Lung 19(4): 373–378

24. Teasdale G, Jennett B (1974) Assessment of coma and impaired consciousness: a practical scale. Lancet, ii, 81–84

25. van der Kamp LJT, Bijleveld CCJH (1998) Methodological issues in longitudinal research. In: Longitudinal data analysis: designs, models and methods, In: Bijleverd CCJH, van der Kamp LJ, Mooijaart A, van der Kloot WA, van der Leeden R, van der Burg E (eds) Sage Publications, London, p 1–45

26. Van Woerkom TCAM, Minderhoud JM, Gottschal T, Nicolai G (1982) Neurotransmitters in the treatment of patients with severe head injuries. Eur Neurol 21: 227–234

27. Von Wild K, Simons P, Schoeppner H (1992) Effect of pyritinol on EEG and SSEP in comatose patients in the acute phase of intensive care therapy. Pharmacopsychiatry 25(3): 157–165

28. Wood RL, Winkowski TB, Miller JL, Tierney L, Goldman L (1992) Evaluating sensory regulation as a method to improve awareness in patients with altered states of consciousness: a pilot study. Brain Inj 6(5): 411–418

Correspondence: M. Vanier, Université de Montréal, Québec, Canada.

Acta Neurochir (2001) [Suppl] 79: 59–60

What is a Good Re-Entry Programme? What are the Key-Question? – *J. Douglas Miller Memorial Lecture*

D. N. Brooks

Rehab without Walls, Crownhill, Milton Keynes, UK

What does it take to make a good rehabilitation service? At first sight, this seems a simplistic, even impossible question to answer. After all, rehabilitation is delivered in many different situations, at different times after injury, and by very different groups of people. Furthemore, as rehabilitation professionnals often point out, patients with acquired brain injury (ABI) form a very diverse group with different needs, and there is no one "golden rule" for rehabilitation.

This lecture will argue that the requirements for good ABI rehabilitation are simple (at least, simple to specify), readily available (see CARF) and are no more than a code of conduct that ensures that every ABI patient is given the kind of rehabilitation that every professionnal would want if they had an ABI. Here are some simple rules:

Know Your Population

Yes, ABI patients are a diverse group, but the similitaries are greater than the differences. A knowledge of the typical characteristics of your patients (demographic and clinical) allows you to focus your effort on achievable clinical goals.

Have a Treatment Plan

It is critical to ensure that every patient has a Treatment Plan with clearly defined goals: suggested times to reach those goals; and a mechanism for checking that the goals have been reached, or if not, that appropriate changes in the Plan are made.

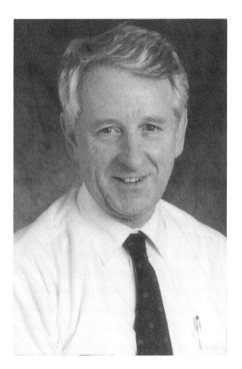

Fig. 1. J. Douglas Miller

Have a Skilled Team

This is easier to specify than to achieve. This is because ABI rehabilitation has expanded in many parts of the world, but the training of specialist staff has not expanded at the same rate. As a result, it is increasingly difficult to find key staff such as Occupational Therapist. If such staff cannot readily be found, then a rehabilitation service MUST consider how to ensure that patients are given skilled service (e.g. the use of external staff consultants, Therapy Aides). The exact skill

---

* CARF: Committee for Accreditation of Rehabilitation Facilities.

mix will depend on the nature of the patients being rehabilitated.

Have "in House" Training and Staff Development

As it may be difficult to find key staff, it is vital to motivate, train, and support the staff that are there in the unit.

A Flexible Team

ABI rehabilitation demands flexible allocation of resources, and the most expensive resource is staff. Members of a team have to be prepared to blur roles. The team must be as stable as possible, as inconsistency is a major cause of deterioration in behaviour of patients.

Leadership

The team must have a determined, knowledgeable, and credible leader. The professionnal background of the leader will depend on the patients being rehabilitated.

Look after the Rights of the Patient

Treat everyone with dignity. For every proposed action or policy, ask how you would feel if you were the patient.

Behaviour

Decide how you will deal with the inevitable behaviour problems that patients will show. Ensure that key staff are trained and experienced in behaviour management.

Acta Neurochir (2001) [Suppl] 79: 61–64

Health Management Technology for Catastrophic Medical Conditions

D. N. Cope, E. D. Bryant, and **P. Sundance**

ParadigmHealth Corporation, California, United States of America

Summary

Background. The excessive growth of health care expenditures in the United States is widely acknowledged. Costs are anticipated to double by the year 2006. The intractable issue which remains before health care leaders is how to appropriately restrain these costs while not sacrificing a desired level of care quality. A variety of management approaches have been developed in pursuit of more rational and cost-effective use of health resources. Current management approaches have proven inadequate in stemming health care cost inflation and have raised increasing concerns about their negative impact on the quality of health care.

Method. One group has created and operated a data and structured, expert consensus-driven health management technology for the management of catastrophic medical conditions, including severe brain and spinal cord injury and severe multiple trauma and burns, since 1992 and has recently applied this same technology to high risk neonates and organ transplants. This integrated, severity risk adjusted, delivery system incorporates adequate clinical data capture and analysis, coupled with empirically derived management principles and consensus expert clinical judgment.

Interpretation. Preliminary data analysis indicates that patients treated under the ParadigmHealth model experienced an improvement in the health care process, improved quality in health care delivery and outcomes, and overall cost reduction.

Keywords: Health management technology; costs of care paradigm health corporation; evidence based care traumatic brain injuries.

Introduction

The excessive growth of health care expenditures in the United States and elsewhere is widely acknowledged, and annual expenditures are anticipated to double by the year 2007 reaching 16.6% of the United States Gross Domestic Product, or 2.1 trillion dollars [1, 2]. The intractable issue, which remains before health care leaders, is how to appropriately restrain these costs while not sacrificing a desired level of care quality. A variety of management approaches have been developed in pursuit of more rational, standardized and cost-effective use of health resources.

Current management approaches have proven inadequate in stemming health care cost inflation and have raised increasing concerns about their negative impact on the quality of health care [3, 4, 5]. Further, there is a low probability that most present techniques can have a significant beneficial impact in the future [6], especially on very complex, costly medical conditions. This paper describes a management approach that has proven successful with a subset of these complex conditions: namely; severe brain and spinal cord injury, severe multiple trauma and burns, and high-risk neonates, and most recently organ transplants. It is proposed that this same model can serve as a template for other complex conditions[a]. We will first briefly review limitations of current medical care management methodologies, and then introduce a new health management technology and structure which represents a novel and powerful methodology to appropriately and rationally achieve cost containment and quality of care.

In the United States, health care today, while of generally high quality, is marked by inconsistent and, at times, inappropriate delivery of services. Commonly, physicians rely upon their own unsystematic clinical observations drawn primarily from personal experience in making treatment decisions. Decisions made and conclusions drawn reflect the unsystematic biases of a given physician and contribute to marked variability in practices among clinicians and to the escalation of medical costs [7, 8]. In addition, the complexity of modern health care, involving co-morbidities, questions of long-term outcomes overlaying short-term acute care management, and complex outcome constructs such as "quality of life" versus solely "biologi-

---

[a] Severe congenital heart defects, pediatric oncology, children with complex multiple needs, AIDS, etc.

cal viability", is itself an impediment to making rational treatment and reimbursement decisions. Evidence-based medicine (EBM) has emerged in an attempt to ground medical decision-making (and by corollary health care funding decisions) in scientifically sound, experimentally based knowledge [9]. Where applicable, EBM is extremely powerful in determining what is or is not "medically" necessary, indicated, or harmful. However, many (if not most), health care interventions have not met (and are unlikely to ever meet) the degree of scientific certainty inherent in EBM. Much of health care is too complex with inadequate data to allow evidence-based decisions. Seemingly straightforward clinical interventions are now understood to have second, third, and fourth order interactions with other outcome determinants that preclude obvious cause and effect conclusions [10].

Given the costs and complexity in the delivery of modern health care, multiple management methodologies have been developed to restrain inappropriate health care and escalating costs: price controls (limiting reimbursement for individual or aggregate services); preferred provider organizations (PPO's-reduced rates from contracted providers in return for an expected increase in volume); utilization review (UR-external review of need for ongoing prescribed services); case management (primarily a nurse UR function without sufficient expertise or power to affect the care process, especially for complex conditions); financial risk-transferring techniques such as diagnosis related group reimbursement (DRGs-provider reimbursement based upon specific diagnostic code); and capitating payment for populations (provider reimbursement based upon a "per member per month" rate of payment regardless of services provided.) While undoubtedly of some effect, these methodologies are widely seen as heavy-handed, arbitrary, and intrusive, such that short-term savings (reflected in reduced premiums for the next annual insurance contract cycle) has become the primary determinant of "success" for health plans. In particular, it has been documented that neither the purchasers nor the providers of health care have developed methods of capitation or delivery which successfully lead to appropriate high quality care for patients with complex chronic or disabling conditions, or conditions of relative infrequency [11, 12, 13, 14].

To summarize, current health care management methods have not been adequately effective either clinically or financially and are widely acknowledged to be heavy-handed, uninformed, arbitrary and inflexible. What effectiveness there is appears to be approaching maximal impact. In addition, they are increasingly aversive to the patient and practicing physician, and are in many instances harmful to quality care, particularly so for the most complex conditions. These changes in health care have produced a highly charged, emotional milieu with lack of a general consensus on how to rationally and fairly approach these cost-quality dilemmas.

Methods and Results

A Prototype Solution

In response to the evident deficiencies of early management efforts as well as the enormous costs associated with both short and long term treatment of complex conditions (first year costs over a million dollars per case for the severest conditions), it is critical that a new management system be implemented that incorporates adequate clinical data capture and analysis, coupled with empirically derived management principles (including but not limited to EBM). Such a system must also recognize the limitations of a purely data and science driven management approach, and integrate these where necessary with a structured approach based upon consensus expert clinical judgment. For the past eight years the authors have participated in the development of such a system at ParadigmHealth Corporation (PHC). The model incorporates a technology of health management for complex conditions which makes systematic use of many newer methodologies such as evidence-based medicine, Ellwood's concept of a "technology of patient experience" [15], (i.e. the comprehensive capture and analysis of large clinical and economic data sets which characterize the treatment pattern and outcomes of complex conditions longitudinally over prolonged periods), virtual integrated delivery systems, capitation based upon appropriate risk-adjustment, comprehensive process and outcomes measurements, application of medical expertise by qualified physician specialists, and others.

PHC's model is designed to ensure that each provider along the continuum of complex care has the necessary expertise to identify and address the appropriate clinical problem(s) with the most efficient resource consumption in order to provide the optimal clinical outcome. To do so, PHC assigns a core team of experts to each case. The critical members of this Complex Medical Event Management Team (CMT) include physician specialists, specialist nurse network managers (NWMs), and directors of clinical service (DCSs). The specialist physician medical directors (PMDs) and medical specialist consultants (MSCs) are practicing specialist physicians across the United States under contractual arrangement with PHC who provide high level clinical expertise for assessment of current problems, identifying reasonable target outcomes, planning of continuum of care strategies, projections of appropriate resources, and proactive management interventions. They are board certified physicians in one or more medical and/or surgical specialties with a practice expertise and focus appropriate to the management of the diagnostic categories assigned. The NWMs are registered nurses with extensive case management expertise, particularly in the management of complex injury, most of whom have earned advanced degrees and certification in the fields of rehabilitation, critical care nursing, neonatal nursing, and case management. These NWMs are under contractual arrangement with PHC and work within close proximity of the patient so that they can provide on-site independent assessment and management. The DCSs are PHC employees with years of training and experience in medical-clinical resource utilization and risk management with advanced clinical degrees and certifications. They have the primary accountability for integrating database measures encompassing empirical clinical and economic information on large samples of similar severity adjusted cases (see below) into a specific outcome plan and budget for each new case and for directing the management of that case to its completion.

In addition to having an expert driven management team, PHC's model also considers it essential to have providers and facilities that have the clinical expertise to treat such highly complex patients. Identifying these providers can be a significant challenge. For example, Joint Commission on Accreditation of Healthcare Organizations (JCAHO) certification does not necessarily ensure a facility's capacity to provide top-quality care for highly complex problems. The concept of centers of excellence (COE) to identify facilities with such diagnosis or condition-specific capabilities arose in response to this issue and PHC identifies, qualifies, and contracts with premier providers (COEs). Frequently, difficulty exists moving patients from local facilities to regionally based COEs (some located a considerable distance from the patient's home and families). In these circumstances PHC applies high levels of medical expertise "at a distance" via electronic consultations between the CMT and the attending clinicians. Overall, PHC creates a capability to manage very complex patient care and recovery across the continuum of care, providing oversight, access to data on outcomes of various treatment choices, and a broader level of expertise to its program providers (especially attending physicians), allowing appropriate allocation of resources, and greater understanding of total costs compared to traditional systems. By feeding this information back to physicians, facilities and health administrators Paradigm provides a powerful foundation for understanding the consequences of care decisions for complex medicine. PHC contributes to the health care process, following Eddy's suggestion,

"The solution [to practice variability] is not to remove the decision-making power from physicians, but to improve the capacity of physicians to make better decisions. To achieve this solution, we must give physicians the information they need; we must institutionalize the skills to use that information; and we must build processes that support, not dictate, decisions [16]."

To provide such information, education, advice, and economic incentives to all providers of care (and to payers where appropriate), and to measure performance against norms, it is imperative that a comprehensive database be used, one that is designed to capture information at injury/illness onset and throughout the entire course of care, including intervals after recovery is complete. Measurements must include prediction, process, and outcome variables. PHC has established such an objective database that allows for meaningful analysis of the effect of various pathways of care by various providers upon objective outcomes of appropriately risk-adjusted populations of complex medical patients (appropriate Severity Risk Adjustment "SRA" is applied to each complex medical condition PHC manages). This database is kept in an electronic relational format that allows complex statistical analyses to be effectively performed.

Inherent in the PHC databased model is the identification of appropriate clinical outcomes and the measurement of these outcomes to determine if in fact they have been achieved. Health care driven by appropriate outcomes has a variety of benefits. It allows patients in any phase of treatment, from acute injury or illness through complete reintegration into society and work, to be operationally described and classified [17] or grouped. It thus serves as a foundation

upon which specific treatment interventions can be arranged and evaluated regarding appropriateness of resource utilization (both expected and actual). Paradigm has developed clinical outcome definitions that are objective and meaningful to all the stake holders of complex conditions, i.e. the patients, the providers and the payers. These operational outcomes set the foundation for a system of communication and accountability for the stake holders, upon which financial and operational contractual agreements can operate.

To meet the above data requirements while still achieving statistically significant conclusions, it is necessary to have a great number of cases. As a practical matter, this requires a data set from a very large population of lives at risk, essentially a nationally based collection. Paradigm operates nationally to collect objective, comparable data that can meet this volume requirement. This allows as well the capacity to measure and do comparisons on regional variations in care provision, processes of care, relevant outcome, and cost. Thus, for example, the observed fact that some regions of the country have much shorter in-patient treatment stays for brain and spinal injuries, burns and high-risk neonates could be interpreted as representing either appropriate cost efficiency or inappropriate withholding of care. PHC is able to use objective clinical and financial analysis rather than subjective opinion to make this determination. In addition, as advances in care are introduced by any provider in a complex care system, it can quickly and virtually "automatically" be compared with results already achieved by conventional methods by other providers and informed decisions can then be made about cost-benefit.

Discussion

The escalation in health care costs as well as current medical practice that lacks both scientific rigor and fiscal accountability are increasingly recognized as limitations inherent in traditional medical management. Data driven management has emerged as a new strategy in health care management. According to some observers, these changes in health care and medical practice reflect nothing less than a true paradigm shift for our health care system. For nearly a decade, PHC has integrated these strategies and applied them with measurable success to complex medical conditions, which characteristically represent the most clinically difficult and costly problems in medicine. The PHC system has done so for over 4400 such cases in its eight years of clinical operation, 1283 of which have been cases of severe traumatic brain injury. In each of these managed cases specific objective and auditable clinical and financial outcomes were achieved and measured. A variety of evidence has suggested that these outcomes and costs are significantly improved over non-PHC managed cases of equal complexity. More methodologically complete investigations are currently underway to quantify these results. The authors believe the systematic construction and organization of this system, as well as its demonstrated generalizability, make it of international interest to all medical and health policy readers. The elements and construction of this system in its entirety constitutes a new management paradigm for health care.

References

1. Smith S, Freeland M, Heffler S, McKusick D *et al* (1998) The next ten years of health spending: what does the future hold? Health Affairs 17(5): 128–140

2. Smith S, Heffler S, Freeland M *et al* (1998) The next decade of health spending: a new outlook. Health Affairs 18(4): 86–95

3. Schwartz William B (1998) Life without disease: the pursuit of medical utopia. University of California Press, Berkeley, California, pp 92–94

4. Mechanic D (1997) Managed care as a target of distrust. JAMA, June 11, 277(22): 1810–1811

5. Jenkins Jr HW (2000) Managed care meets its maker. Wall Street Journal, February 23

6. Ginzberg E (1997) Managed care and the competitive market in health care: what they can and cannot do. JAMA, June 11, 277(22): 1812–1813

7. Walters BC (1998) Clinical practice parameter development in neurosurgery. In: Bean J (ed) Neurosurgery in transition. Williams & Wilkins, Baltimore, MD, pp 99–106

8. Walters BC (1998) Clinical practice parameter development in neurosurgery. In: Bean J (ed) Neurosurgery in transition. Williams & Wilkins, Baltimore, MD, pp 99–106

9. Eddy DM (1996) Clinical decision making: from theory to practice. Jones and Bartlett Publishers, Sudbury, MA, pp 6–7

10. Horn SC, Sharkey PD, Tracy DM, Horn CE, James B, Goodwin F (1996) Intended and unintended consequences of HMO cost-containment strategies: results from the managed care outcomes project. Am J Managed Care 11(3): 253–264

11. Sutton J, DeJong G (1998) Managed care and people with disabilities: framing the issues. Arch Phys Med Rehab 79: 1312–1316

12. Kuhlthau K, Walker D, Perrin J *et al* (1998) Assessing managed care for children with chronic conditions. Health Affairs 17(4): 42–52

13. Sandy L, Gibson R (1996) Managed care and chronic care: challenges and opportunities. Managed Care Qu 4(2): 5–11

14. Tanenbaum S, Hurley R (1995) Disability and the managed care frenzy: a cautionary note. Health Affairs 14(4): 213–219

15. Ellwood P (1988) Special report: Shattuck lecture – outcomes management. A technology of patient experience. NEJM, June 9, 318(1): 549–1556

16. Eddy DM (1996) Clinical decision making: from theory to practice. Jones and Bartlett Publishers, Sudbury, MA, p 8

17. Cope N, Sundance P (1995) Conceptualizing clinical outcomes. In: Landrum P *et al* (ed) Outcome oriented rehabilitation: principals, strategies, and tools for effective program management. Aspen Publishers, Gaithersburg, MD, pp 43–56

Correspondence: D. Nathan Cope, M.D., ParadigmHealth Corporation, 1001 Galaxy Way, Suite 300, Concord, California 94520, United States of America.

Part II: Functional Neurosurgery and Neuromodulation

Acta Neurochir (2001) [Suppl] 79: 67–74

The Important Role of Pain in Neurorehabilitation. The Neurosurgeon's Approach Or (Neurorehabilitation: The Neurosurgeon's Role with Special Emphasis on Pain and Spasticity)

C. A. Pagni, S. Canavero, V. Bonicalzi, and C. Nurisso

Neurosurgical Clinic, University of Torino, Italy

Summary

Pain syndromes due to peripheral or central nervous system damage, or both, may hinder neurorehabilitation. Control of pain may be obtained by ablative or augmentative procedures. Of the ablative modes only DREZ and Cordectomy are still being employed in cases of pain due to Brachial Plexus Avulsion and conus and cauda damage at T9-L1: in both pain is not simply due to "deafferentation". The augmentative procedures include spinal cord, deep brain and cortical stimulation. Subarachnoid infusion of drugs (midazolam, clonidine, baclofen, etc.) is a new avenue open to control pain.

Indications, results and mechanisms of action of those procedures in neuropathic pain are discussed on the basis of literature and personal experience.

Keywords: Neurorehabilitation; pain relief, neurosurgery, ablative and augmentative procedures.

Introduction

Control of pain is one of man's basic needs and has been approached over the centuries by both rational and superstitious means.

Chronic incapacitating pain is often arbitrarily divided into cancer pain and non-cancer pain, which is frequently initiated or caused by a primary lesion or dysfunction in the peripheral or central nervous system (neurogenic or neuropathic pain and central pain) (Turk DC, Okifuji A, 2001). Injury to peripheral nervous system produces pain by both abnormal persistent afferent discharges (augmented, as Claude Bernard maintained) in damaged nerves, and denervation with ensuing central nervous system function derangement [10]. Pain secondary to central nervous system (CNS) injury, either to the brain itself or to the spinal cord, is defined as central pain (CP). However, many other non-malignant diseases (for example chronic arthritis and arthrosis) can also produce chronic pain, which is poorly responsive to standard treatments.

Surgical management of non-cancer pain is a major undertaking that should be considered only when the pain interferes enough with the patient's quality of life and more conservative measures have failed or produce unacceptable side effects to justify the risk associated with surgery.

In planning a management for chronic refractory pain the patient's complaints and the characters of the pain should be documented and differentiated; the etiology, the origin and, possibly, the pathophysiology of the patient's symptoms should be accurately explained, also including pharmacologic dissection. Pharmacologic dissection allows identification of nociceptive (fentanyl test), neuropathic (lidocaine test) or central components (propofol test), which warrants different therapeutic strategies [2].

In fact, in certain syndromes, generally labelled as CP, different mechanisms giving rise to different kinds of pain may be at work, as e.g. central and peripheral mechanisms in pain in paraplegics due to injury at T9–T10 level [3].

So, depending on the suspected problem, specific investigations might be useful; for example, a patient suffering from failed back surgery syndrome (FBSS) who is being considered for dorsal column stimulation deserves at least radiographs with flexion extension, a contrasted MRI and sufficient laboratory studies to rule out a residual or recurrent disc fragment, instability or subclinical infection.

Psychiatric evaluation allows identifying secondary gain issue or psychopathology which may amount to a contraindication for surgery. Psychological evaluation may also help to define the patient's expectation for outcome. It is mandatory to ensure that the patient understands what the physician expects the procedure to accomplish and what are the risks of the procedure.

It is important to formulate some plan for dealing with patients' narcotic intake and this must be clarified with the patient before surgery.

The neurosurgeon is called into service for the following pain syndromes which may hinder neurorehabilitation:

1) Pain following peripheral nervous system injuries including nerve roots (*peripheral neuropathic pain*)
2) Pain following central nervous system injuries (*central pain*)
3) Mixed complex pains due to both central and peripheral mechanisms, which also may include a peripheral nociceptive component, such as paraplegia pain following vertebral fractures at T9-L1 damaging both the cord and the cauda.

Surgical Techniques for non Malignant Pain

Surgical techniques for non malignant pain can generally be classified as neuroablative or neuroaugmentative. Neuroablative procedures are based on the concept that transection of neural pathways that normally carry nociceptive input in the peripheral (e.g. neurectomy, rhizotomy) or central nervous system (e.g. anterolateral cordotomy, ventroposterolateral-ventroposteromedial thalamotomy, (VPL-VPM)) should eliminate that input and consequently eliminate pain. Transection of sensory pathways usually relieves, at least for a short period, pain, but sometimes it is followed by recurrences or development of an even worse pain, for instance, anaesthesia dolorosa, postcordotomy dysesthesia, central pain [10].

Neuroaugmentative or modulatory procedures, on the other hand, rely on the ability of the central nervous system to manipulate or modify sensory input. Therapeutic use of this notion began following the introduction of the gate control theory of pain and the discovery of inhibitory descending pathways controlling pain input [8]. Examples of augmentative procedures are chronic stimulation of the dorsal columns or deep brain structures and intraspinal drug delivery.

We shall focus our report on surgical procedures both ablative and augmentative which may be employed in neuropathic and/or central pain.

Ablative Procedures

Out of the armamentarium summarized on Table 1, the still useful weapons for certain kinds of central and/or neuropathic pain are *DREZ* and *cordomyelotomy*. Cordotomy, stereotactic thalamotomy and mesencephalotomy are only exceptionally employed [10].

Cordotomy, i.e. the section of the neospinothalamic tract, was the most employed ablative procedure for pain relief especially for cancer pain. In spite of the fact that there is a small number of patients that underwent cordotomy years ago for nociceptive non cancer pain who have a persisting analgesia and no new pain, experience has demonstrated that cordotomy can result, in those cases, in a new, if not worse, pain syndrome: postcordotomy dysesthesia. For instance, no more than 30% of paraplegics was permanently relieved by cordotomy [13].

Thalamotomy consists in creating stereotactic lesions in the VPL-VPM, center median, parafascicular

Table 1. *Surgical Procedures for Relief of Pain*

Ablative
Peripheral
– Intrathecal alcohol, phenol, cold saline infusions
– Neurectomy
– Sympathectomy, e.g., for pancreatic pain
– Posterior rhizotomy
– Ganglionectomy

Central
– Dorsal root entry zone lesion (DREZ)
– Anterolateral cordotomy
– Myelotomy, cordectomy, cordomyelotomy
– Trigeminal tractotomy and nucleotomy
– Medullary tractotomy
– Pontine tractotomy
– Mesencephalic tractotomy
– Various thalamotomy techniques (VPL-VPM, CM, intralaminar, parafascicular)
– Procedures on thalamic radiations and cortex
– Cingulotomy
– Hypothalamotomy

Other
– Operations on hypophysis, including intrasellar alcohol injection

Augmentative and modulatory
– Epidural, intrathecal, intraventricular infusions: morphine, midazolam, clonidine and others
– Thalamic, internal capsule stimulation
– Periaquaeductal/periventricular gray (PVG/PAG) stimulation
– Dorsal column stimulation
– Cortical stimulation
– Hypothalamic stimulation

and intralaminar nuclei and also in the pulvinar. These nuclei are believed to receive input from the specific pain pathways (VPL-VPM) and the protopathic portion of the spinothalamic system which reaches the thalamus after polysynaptic relay in the midbrain periaquaeductal reticular formation. Satisfactory pain relief following thalamotomy tends to be short-lived so the use of this procedure is justified in case of failure of alternative medical and surgical modalities [10].

Dorsal root entry zone (DREZ) coagulation in the spinal cord is indicated for pain secondary to brachial plexus avulsion or lumbosacral plexus avulsion. It is also indicated for the relief of end-zone pain associated with spinal cord injury.

The rationale for DREZ was, according to its proponent, Dr. Nashold, that pain in brachial plexus avulsion and paraplegia is a pure form of deafferentation pain: deafferented hyperactive dorsal horn secondary nociceptive neurons generate pain. The aim of DREZ is to destroy the pain generator.

We proposed a more elaborate mechanism of action [11].

Brachial plexus avulsion (BPA) is usually incomplete, involving parts of the rootlets, and most patients suffering from pain have an incomplete sensory loss. Also, the plexus is involved elsewhere as well. Damaged fibers of incompletely avulsed roots and plexus may present neuromas at injury site. These are the favorite sites of ectopic pacemakers, which are highly sensitive to mechanical distorsion, changes in temperature, potassium, ischemia, sympathetic activity, catecholamines and whose activity may be increased by "cross-talking". Afferent impulses originating from such ectopic pacemakers may sustain brachial plexus avulsion pain. Following peripheral nerve injury, dorsal horn multimodal neurons expand their receptive fields and denervation leads to reduction of the center-surround inhibitory mechanism of tactile receptive fields. Touch stimuli will then activate a larger number of multimodal neurons in the peripheral zones of their receptive fields and produce activity in the central ascending pathways mimicking that normally induced by noxious stimuli: this hyperexcitability may be perceived as increased pain. That may also explain the occurrence of trigger zones at the periphery of denervated dermatomes, whose activation increases pain. This mechanism may be responsible for pain paroxysms and may also activate metameric interneurons as well and, hence, anterior horn motoneurons, with ensuing spasms and twitches (rarely seen in BPA, as the

anterior motor roots are more likely to be torn off than the posterior ones) [10].

A similar mechanism is also at the origin of so-called end-zone pain due to traumatic lesions at the thoracolumbar passage (T10-L1), which involve both the cord lumbar enlargement and cauda roots with formation of neuromas [12] but also other levels. In cord injuries, pathologically active multimodal cells found in damaged cord or below the injury level, whose receptive fields are linked to partially or apparently totally denervated body regions, may still be connected to upper centers by damaged fibers, which can but transmit improperly coded impulses. As in brachial plexus avulsion, their activity will mimick pain, which may also be paroxysmal: pain will be referred with a radicular-like distribution onto large areas of altered sensation or to seemingly totally denervated areas. Spasms may also be present, as in BPA (Fig. 1).

The best results with DREZ have been reported in patients with BPA and in cases of conus medullaris root avulsion, more then 70% being relieved from pain [7, 10].

DREZ proved effective in pain due to traumatic lesions at T9-L1 involving the conus medullaris and cauda equina. Most of these patients have end-zone pain, with constant aching and burning pain, together with paroxysms of pain (cramping, stabbing, electrical) referred to hypesthetic areas, often with incomplete neurological deficits and associated muscle spasms. About 70% have a satisfactory relief from pain after a mean follow-up of 3 years. However, the complication rate may be as high as 30% and includes motor and sphincteric deficits, particularly in patients with spinal cord damage and in those who underwent bilateral DREZ lesions. Importantly, patients with diffuse burning and dysesthetic pain, below the level of the cord lesion, worst or limited to the sacral region, are usually not relieved from pain.

Cordectomies and cordomyelotomies have been seldom employed. However, persistent relief has been obtained usually of pain due to lesions at and below the T10–11 vertebral level with resection at or around the T10–11 level, including ablation of the cauda. Results are less rewarding with lesions and section at higher cord levels. Best results are reported for patients complaining of shooting, paroxysmal pain and spasms [12]. For cordectomy too, pain referred to the lower abdomen, and burning or dysesthetic pain diffused to the legs or localized to the buttocks or feet usually has not been relieved [10]. Cordectomy (as DREZ) in high

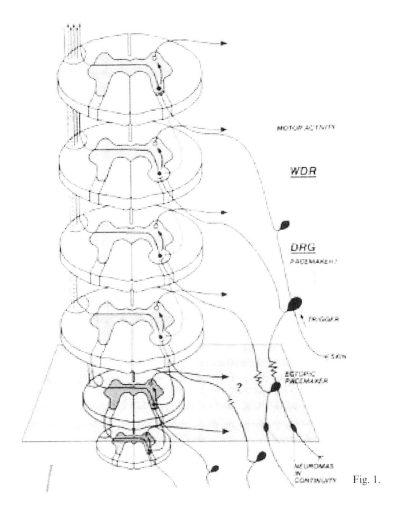

Fig. 1.

thoracic lesions may relieve girdle pain (end-zone pain) and paroxysmal pain, leaving diffuse burning pain unchanged.

In sum, the good results of DREZ surgery and cordectomy on end-zone pain in such kinds of lesions depend on the pain not being simply due to "deafferentation", but to active mechanisms: these are extinguished or blocked by destruction of dorsal horns or ablation of damaged cord and roots or switched off by any ascending connections [11, 12]. Dysesthesias and eventual burning in the legs and perineum (so called diffuse pain) are usually refractory to demolitive procedures. The latter are likely due to anomalous processing in the thalamus and cortex [4].

At this time, DREZ lesions can be applied in well-defined pains at the level of a spinal lesion and cordectomies should be considered more often in pain with paraplegia. DREZ surgery is the operation of choice for end zone or segmental pain in a paraplegic,

and the relief can be expected to last for long periods of time, i.e. five years or more. Certainly, cordectomies relieve the same types of pain that respond to cordotomy [10].

A common complaint hindering rehabilitation is pain in chronic cervical spondylosis. Pain may be due to radicular compression in the foramina and referred to the upper limbs and shoulder and to cervical myelopathy and referred to arms, torso, and legs.

Radicular pain may be treated with permanent relief by foraminotomy or less frequently by an anterior approach; foraminotomy can be performed also at multiple level and bilaterally.

Pain in chronic myelopathy, due to the stenosis of the cervical spinal canal, usually observed in patients with a hyperintense signal in T2 at Magnetic Resonance, does not subside after cervical decompression by anterior or posterior approaches.

Very rarely CP with hyperalgesia develops early

after cervical injury in spondylothic spine, owing to irritative mechanisms: it is relieved by surgical decompression [3].

Augmentative Surgery

Transcutaneous Electrical Nerve Stimulation (TENS). TENS, whose mechanism of action remains poorly understood, is employed for pain due to BPA, central nervous system damage and spinal cord lesion with variable results [10]. Usually it cannot be relied upon as a definitive approach.

Spinal Cord Stimulation (SCS). Spinal cord stimulation (dorsal column stimulation) has been attempted in various kinds of neuropathic pain due to peripheral lesions, CP due to brain and spinal cord damage, phantom and amputation pain. Results are highly variable: it seems not indicated in CP of brain and cord origin and in complete BPA [10].

This modality is useful for treating residual radicular pain following disk surgery that has been at least anatomically successful; the radicular component of postlaminectomy pain is presumably neurophatic in origin. The results of this modality of treatment compare favorably with those of reoperation. Spinal cord stimulation also deserves consideration in the syndrome previously termed reflex sympathetic dystrophy, or complex regional pain syndrome Type I [8].

Deep Brain Stimulation (DBS). In the late 1970s a number of clinical studies provided evidence that intracerebral stimulation, usually referred to as deep brain stimulation (DBS), might be a reliable method for the management of pain otherwise resistant to any therapeutic modality.

DBS has evolved along two lines, corresponding to the two major target regions for stimulation: sensory thalamic nuclei (ventral posterior lateral and medial thalamic nucleus) and posterior limb of the capsula, or periaqueductal-periventricular gray region (PAG/PVG). Conceivably, stimulation in these two regions may influence pain by the activation of different mechanisms and/or systems. There is robust evidence that stimulation in the sensory thalamus is selectively effective for neuropathic pain, whereas PAG/PVG stimulation appears to affect preferentially nociceptive forms of pain.

However, many of the ensuing long-term follow-up studies failed to confirm the first optimistic reports, particularly with regard to the efficacy of the treatment for neuropathic forms of pain [10]. Although DBS has been in use for more than two decades, there are still discordant opinions as to the indications, the preferred stimulation targets, incidence of tolerance and possible countermeasures, biochemical mechanisms involved, and so forth. Most neurosurgeons ceased to practice DBS because they only rarely found a good indication and considered the outcome unpredictable or had themselves often failed to obtain satisfactory results.

Even though it is an invasive procedure, it carries a relatively small risk of complications and side effects.

The efficacy of stimulation in either of the targets is quite variable, ranging from 30% to 80%. In a thorough metaanalysis of all studies including more than 15 patients (13 studies comprising 1114 patients [9]), the long-term good results varied between 19% and 79%. The incidence of favorable overall results decreased during the first year, and for example, Richardson reported a gradual reduction of good results with PAG/PVG stimulation, from 85% to 65%.

In most of the series the longer the follow-up the less the success rate which in neuropathic pain approaches 30%, a rate close to the level of a placebo effect [10].

In the most recent studies it was concluded that low back pain is the best indication for DBS. With PAG/PVG stimulation, and in a few cases with dual electrodes (electrodes both in PAG/PVG and in sensory thalamus), 71% (35 out of 49 patients) reported excellent or good pain relief (more than 50%), considerable reduction of analgesic intake, and improvement in work tolerance. Apart from low back pain, with or without radiating leg pain as a sign of lumbosacral rhizopathy necessitating dual-electrode implantation, the number of patients in each diagnostic group of neuropathic pain is too small to permit any definite conclusions concerning the efficacy of DBS. The possibility that PAG/PVG stimulation may be efficacious also for neuropathic pain has been reported here and there.

On the other hand, sensory thalamic stimulation seems to be completely ineffective for nociceptive forms of pain, and the results are extremely variable also for the different types of neuropathic pain. For example, anesthesia dolorosa is reported to respond favorably in many studies, whereas in others it is concluded that this diagnosis is a bad indication. The results in CP, generally referred to as thalamic pain as well as pain in spinal cord injury are unsatisfactory and these are not generally considered indications for DBS anymore.

DBS has been replaced by extradural cortical stimulation.

Motor Cortex Stimulation (MCS). In recent years, stimulation of the precentral motor area (Brodman 4) applied via a four-pole stimulating electrode placed epidurally has attracted much interest. This treatment, which was introduced by Tsubokawa in 1989, has proven to be efficient particularly for central poststroke pain. Moreover, motor cortex stimulation (MCS) appears to be a promising treatment for painful trigeminal neuropathy, including facial anesthesia dolorosa and perhaps also other forms of pain due to peripheral nerve injury. MCS has been in use for approximately 8 years; however, the underlying mechanisms of its pain-relieving effect are poorly understood, and there are few experimental data pertaining to its mode of action. Mechanisms at work might include: a) suppression of increased neuronal spontaneous discharge of deafferented thalamic and or trigeminal neurons by motor and sensory cortex stimulation, motor cortex being reciprocally connected with sensory cortex, and posterior thalamic nuclei; b) activation of corticofugal inhibitory pathways; c) restoration of deficient inhibitory pain control due to the cerebral lesion causing central pain; d) rebalancing of abnormal signaling between cortex and thalamus. In a case of parietal cortex hypoperfusion, demonstrated with single photon emission computed tomography, MCS produced normalization of the regional cortical circulation and suppression of pain [1].

The most common indications for MCS are CP due to to supraspinal lesion (hemorrhage or infarction), and painful trigeminal neuropathy, including facial anesthesia dolorosa. Occasional cases of pain after cervical root avulsion, pain in paraplegia or tetraplegia, as well as pain after peripheral nerve injury or syringomyelia have been reported, but the number of patients with each of these diagnoses is too small to permit complete evaluation. The overall positive results vary between approximately 45% and 75% of permanently implanted patients.

Some patients with CP report the presence of paroxysmal, shooting pain components besides the deep, aching, and sometimes burning type of spontaneous, continuous pain. It has been reported that also the former intermittent type of pain may be effectively alleviated by MCS. Also, the evoked pain components may be markedly relieved by MCS.

Moreover, MCS applied for trigeminal neuropathy tends to provide somewhat better results than in cases of central pain. The alternative treatments in this condition are stimulation of the trigeminal ganglion/rootlets or sensory thalamic stimulation. Sensory thalamic stimulation often fails, at least in a long-term perspective. For these reasons it is probable that MCS will become the treatment of choice for trigeminal neuropathy [9].

Our experience with 14 patients with neurogenic pain confirms these data [2] (Fig. 2).

Intraspinal Analgesia. Intraspinal narcotic analgesia can be effective in some forms of neural injury pain that are clearly narcotic-responsive. This modality should be used with caution in patients with a normal life expectancy, as the chronic effects of drug administration remain to be determined. In some cases minor interventions are required for equipment malfunction, catheter obstruction, migration, or fracture, and patients become dependent upon a mechanical device for a very long time indeed. A gradual decline in effectiveness over time and drug tolerance development can be observed in a number of patients. There are, however, many patients who seem to maintain a prolonged (years) acceptable level of pain relief using a relatively stable drug infusion rate. Selection criteria to identify these patients remain to be defined.

Central pain appears to be refractory to opioids [10]. On the other hand, infusions of alternative pharmacological agents – anesthetic agents, GABA agonists such as midazolam and baclofen, SNX 111, NMDA antagonists, clonidine – is being actively investigated.

In our experience, 30 patients with central and neuropathic pain have been variously studied with intrathecal midazolam, baclofen, clonidine and morphine. Some excellent results have been observed with long-term infusion [2].

Neurosurgery for Spasticity

Spasticity is one of the most common sequelae of neurologic disease. In most patients, spasticity is useful in compensating for lost motor strength. Nevertheless, in a significant number of patients, it may become excessive and harmful leading to further functional losses.

When uncontrollable by physical therapy, medications and/or botulinum toxin injections, spasticity can benefit from neurostimulation, intrathecal pharmacotherapy or selective ablative procedures. Because excessive hypertonia must be reduced without suppression of the useful muscular tone or impairment in the residual motor and sensory functions, neuroablative procedures must be as selective as possible. These se-

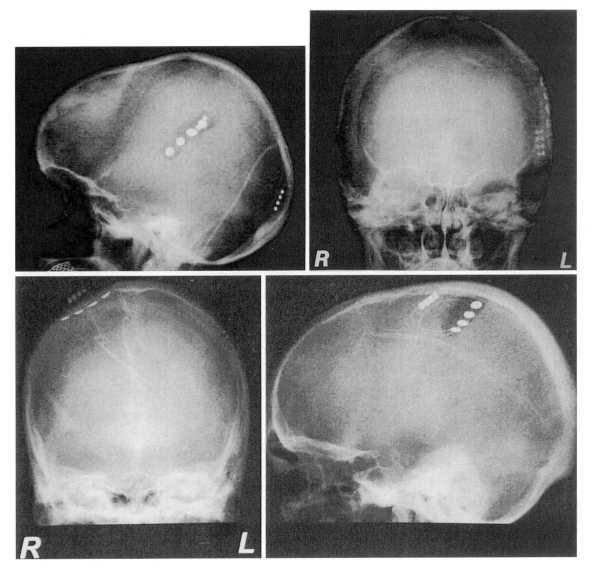

Fig. 2. Extradural cortical stimulators for neurogenic pain in place

lective lesions can be performed at the level of peripheral nerves, spinal roots, spinal cord, or the dorsal root entry zone (DREZ lesions).

In adults, intrathecal baclofen administration is indicated for para- or tetraplegic patients with severe and diffuse spasticity, especially when from spinal origin. Because of its reversibility, this method should be considered prior to any ablative procedure. However, the range between excessive hypotonia with loss of strength and an insufficient effect is very narrow. An intrathecal test through a temporary access port can be useful before permanent implantation.

Neuroablative techniques are indicated for severe localized spasticity in the limbs of paraplegic, tetraplegic or hemiplegic patients.

Neurotomies are preferred when spasticity is localized to muscle groups innervated by a small number of, or a single, peripheral nerve (or nerves). When spasticity affects an entire limb, microsurgical DREZtomy is preferred. Several types of neuroablative procedures can be combined in the treatment of one patient, when needed.

At the Neurosurgical Clinic of Torino, so-called selective posterior rhizotomy has been employed in 27 cases of spasticity due to perinatal encephalopathy with rewarding results in the young.

Whatever the situation and the etiology may be, orthopedic surgery must be considered only after spasticity has been reduced by physical and pharmacological treatments and, when necessary, by neurosurgical procedures.

The general rule is to tailor individual treatments as carefully as possible to the particular problems of the patients.

By suppressing excessive spasticity, correcting abnormal postures, and relieving the frequently associated pain, surgery for spasticity allows physiotherapy to be resumed and sometimes results in the reappearance or improvement of useful voluntary motility. When dealing with these patients, the surgeon must know the risks of the available treatments. To minimize those risks, the surgeon needs a strong anatomic, physiological, and chemical background, rigorous methods to assess and quantify the disorders, and the ability to work in a multidisciplinary team [6].

References

1. Canavero S, Bonicalzi V (1995) Cortical stimulation for central pain. J Neurosurg 83: 117
2. Canavero S, Bonicalzi V (1998) The neurochemistry of central pain: evidence from clinical studies, hypothesis and therapeutic implications (review). Pain 74: 109–114
3. Canavero S, Pagni CA, Bonicalzi V (1995) Transient hyperacute allodynia in Schneider's Syndrome: an irritative genesis. Ital J Neurol Sci 16: 555–557
4. Canavero S, Pagni CA, Castellano G, Bonicalzi V (1994) SPECT and central pain (letter). Pain 57: 129–131
5. Canavero S, Bonicalzi V, Pagni CA, Zeme S, Montrucchio N, Perozzo P (1998) Cortical stimulation for pain; the Turin experience. Proc 4th Intern Congress of the International Neuromodulation Society, 16–20 Sept 1998, Lucerna, Swizerland. Fp 36
6. Gildenberg PL, Tasker RR (eds) (1998) Textbook of stereotactic and functional neurosurgery. McGraw-Hill, New York
7. Gybels JM, Sweet WH (1989) Neurosurgical treatment of persistent pain. In: Gildenberg PL (ed) Pain and headache. Karger, Basel
8. Loeser JD *et al* (eds) (2001) Bonica's management of pain, 3rd edn. Lippincott Williams and Wilkins, Philadelphia
9. Meyerson BA, Linderoth B (2001) Brain stimulation: intracerebral and motor cortex stimulation. In: Loeser JD *et al* (eds) Bonica's management of pain, 3rd edn. Lippincott Williams and Wilkins, Philadelphia, pp 1877–1889
10. Pagni CA (1998) Central pain. A neurosurgical challenge. Edizioni Minerva Medica, Torino
11. Pagni CA, Canavero S (1993) Pain, muscle spasms and twitching fingers following brachial plexus avulsion. Report of three cases relieved by dorsal root entry zone coagulation. J Neurol 240: 468–470
12. Pagni CA, Canavero S (1995) Cordomyelotomy in the treatment of paraplegia pain. Experience in two cases with long-term results. Acta Neurol Belg 95: 33–36
13. White JC, Sweet WH (1969) Pain and the neurosurgeon. A forty-year experience. Thomas CC, Springfield (Ill.)

Correspondence: C. A. Pagni, Neurosurgical Clinic, University of Torino, Italy.

Acta Neurochir (2001) [Suppl] 79: 75–76
© Springer-Verlag 2001

Combined Intrathecal Baclofen and Morphine Infusion for the Treatment of Spasticity Related Pain and Central Deafferentiation Pain

S. Gatscher, R. Becker, E. Uhle, and **H. Bertalanffy**

Department of Neurosurgery, Philipps-University Hospital, Marburg, Germany

Summary

Objectives. Complex pain syndromes due to spasticity and central deafferentation often fail to respond to medical therapy and create challenging problems in the pain management. So far, only spasticity associated musculosceletal pain has been reported to respond to intrathecal baclofen application [1, 2].

Methods. We report the treatment of severe neuropathic pain in a patient with ED and the combined intrathecal application of baclofen and morphine in 5 patients with severe spasticity related pain.

Results. Continous intrathecal baclofen infusion resulted in a pain free period of 20 months in the patient with ED. Patients with spasticity treated with intrathecal application of baclofen and morphine were pain free for a mean period of 2 years.

Conclusion. Intrathecal baclofen and morphin application proved to be effective in spasticity related and central deafferentiation pain and should therefore be considered in the management of these patients.

Keywords: Spasticity; pain; intrathecal baclofen.

Introduction

Complex pain syndromes due to spasticity and central deafferentation often fail to respond to conventional medical therapy and the combination of neurogenic and musculosceletal components create challenging problems in the management of these patients. So far, only spasticity associated musculosceletal pain has been reported to respond to intrathecal baclofen application. We report the successful long-term treatment of severe neuropathic pain in a patient with ED. In addition we describe the combined intrathecal application of baclofen and morphine in 4 patients with severe spasticity where baclofen alone did not achieve sufficient pain relieve. Continuous intrathecal baclofen infusion resulted in a pain free period of 20 months in the patient with ED. Patients with spasticity treated with the intrathecal application of

baclofen and morphine were pain free for a mean period of 2 years. Baclofen alone and in combination with morphine proved to be effective in spasticity related as well as central deafferentiation pain and should therefore be considered in the management of these patients.

Spasticity related pain is in most cases not caused by a single element but by multiple factors. These can be summarised under musculosceletal components and neurogenic components [1, 2]. One component of musculosceletal pain is the increased muscle tonus. If it persists, it will be the origin of irrevocable contractions and secondary joint abnormalities which will again cause spasticity related pain. The neurogenic part of spasticity related pain is, on the other hand, central deafferentiation pain.

Methods

In patients who only suffered from spasticity in its various degrees and not its counteractions good pain control was achieved with intrathecal baclofen only in all cases. If contractions did already exist sufficient pain control could be attained with intrathecal baclofen in most of our patients and morphine was only added in cases with refractory pain syndromes. In the case of joint abnormalities the screening trial was usually started with intrathecal baclofen only, but all of these patients were finally treated with a combined application of intrathecal baclofen and morphine.

In central deafferentiation pain, on the other hand, not only the combination of intrathecal baclofen and morphine, but also individual combinations of baclofen and clonidin have proved to be successful.

Results

Our patient population over the past 5 years consisted of 64 patients who received a medical pump for intrathecal baclofen application at our department. Only 23 patients of this group, however, come to a regular follow-up appointment. The remaining patients are followed up at local hospitals and rehabilitation units where the pumps are also being re-filled.

In the 23 patients who attend our clinic at regular intervals good spasticity and pain regulation was achieved in 19 patients with intrathecal baclofen only. The individual dose required in these patients ranges from 150 to 800 µg per die. In 4 patients we only attained sufficient pain control with a combination of intrathecal baclofen and morphine. The screening trial is usually started with the addition of 20 mg of morphine to 17 ml of baclofen and the morphine dose is then increased until optimal pain control is accomplished in each case. The morphine dose added at each pump filling ranges from 20 to 200 mg MSI. In one patient we only achieved sufficient pain control with a combination of intrathecal baclofen and clonidin. In this patient 0,45 mg of clonidine are added to the baclofen at each pump filling.

Intrathecal baclofen alone or in combination with morphine is, however, also a treatment option in central deafferentiation pain. One of our patients, a 45 year old female who was diagnosed to have MS in 1991, suffered an incomplete spinal cord lesion at TH 5 in 1996 and since then complained of painful paresthesia, dysesthesia and tingeling in both legs. Treated with continuous intrathecal baclofen application via a medical pump this patient achieved complete pain relief for a period of 20 months.

Conclusion

In our experience the combination of intrathecal baclofen and morphin grants good pain control in severe spasticity and its counteractions as well as central deafferentiation pain. In our hand it has not only shown to have a low risk for morbidity but also proved to be an efficient treatment modality. The combination of intrathecal baclofen and morphin or clonidin should therefore be considered in the management of patients with refractory pain syndromes due to spasticity or central deafferentiation pain and should be included in screening trials regularly.

References

1. Loubser PG, Akman NM (1996) Effects of intrathecal baclofen on chronic spinal cord injury pain. J Pain Symptom Manage 12(4): 241–247
2. Middleton JW, Siddall PJ, Walker S, Molloy AR, Rutkowski SB (1996) Intrathecal clonidin and baclofen in the management of spasticity and neuropathic pain following spinal cord injury: a case study. Arch Phys Med Rehabil 77(8): 824–826

Correspondence: S. Gatscher, Department of Neurosurgery, Philipps-University Hospital, Marburg, Germany.

Acta Neurochir (2001) [Suppl] 79: 77–78

The Punctate Midline Myelotomy Concept for Visceral Cancer Pain Control – Case Report and Review of the Literature

R. Becker, S. Gatscher, U. Sure, and H. Bertalanffy

Klinik für Neurochirurgie, Philipps-Universität, Marburg, Germany

Summary

Introduction. Nauta *et al.* first reported on a successful punctate midline myelotomy (PMM) at the spinal cord Th 10 level for the treatment of intractable pelvic cancer pain.

Case Study. The authors published another case history of a patient with multiple anaplastic carcinomas of the small intestine, peritoneal carcinosis and retroperitoneal lymphomas, suffering from severe visceral pain in the hypo-, meso-, and epigastrium. Nauta's PMM was successfully performed at the level Th 4. Narcotic medication was tapered from 30 mg iv. morphine per hour preoperatively to 5 mg per hour within 5 days postoperatively. Pain intensity decreased from 10 to 2–3 on the visual analog scale. Only minor transient side effects appeared postoperatively. Pain reduction remained until the patient died from the extended disease five weeks later.

Discussion. Meanwhile Nauta *et al.* reported on 5 additional patients, in whom PMM led to a sufficient pain reduction. Another paper reported on sufficient control of visceral pain due to advanced stomach cancer after a modified Th 1–2 PMM.

Conclusion. PMM sufficiently controls not only pelvic visceral pain, but also visceral pain generated in the meso- and epigastrium. The findings support the concept of a midline dorsal column visceral pain pathway.

Keywords: Visceral pain; myelotomy; pain pathway.

Introduction

The treatment of visceral pain resulting from either tumour infiltration or therapeutical side effects is one of the major problems in clinical practice. Nauta *et al.* reported about a successful punctate midline myelotomy (PMM) to treat intractable pelvic pain [5]. PMM targets a newly described dorsal column visceral pain pathway that is reported to convey pelvic visceral nociceptive afferents [1, 3]. We reported on a successful PMM in a patient suffering from severe visceral pain, additionally generated in the epi-, and mesogastric region [2]. Meanwhile further reports on successful PMM's appeared and will be reviewed.

Patient and Methods

A 41 year old male had a right upper lobectomy in 4/97, to treat an adenocarcinoma. A few weeks later the patient developed abdominal pain. A diagnostic laparotomy revealed multiple anaplastic carcinomas of the small intestine, peritoneal carcinosis and retroperitoneal lymphomas.

The patient suffered from an excruciating, continuous aching, stabbing, pricking abdominal pain without local preference, nearly unresponsive to medical therapy. With 30 mg/h iv. morphine and high dose metamizole the patient still complained of severe abdominal pain, graded 10 on the visual analog scale (VAS 0–10). Additionally, intermittent colic pain appeared with bowel movements. A coeliac plexus block was rejected with regard to the extended retroperitoneal lymphomas.

It was discussed to proceed with the operation although the pain was not restricted to the hypogastrium. With respect to the extent to the meso- and epigastrium Nauta's PMM was performed at the level Th 4. (Fig. 1 a+b).

Postoperative Course

Immediately after the operation the patient reported about a pain reduction from 10 (VAS) preoperatively to 2–3 postoperatively. The intermittent colic pain had disappeared. The continuous aching, stabbing, pricking pain was reduced to the above mentioned intensity and had lost the stabbing, pricking quality. As neurological complications a transient urinary retention, requiring intermittent catheterization, and paraesthesias in both feet appeared during the first 24 hours after the operation. No other signs of dorsal column dysfunction appeared. Within the first five days of the postoperative course i.v. morphine was reduced to 5 mg/h. A further reduction led to withdrawal symptoms. The patient was discharged five days postoperatively and unfortunately died 5 weeks later from the extended disease. However, he had a significant improvement of his pain and quality of life, until he died.

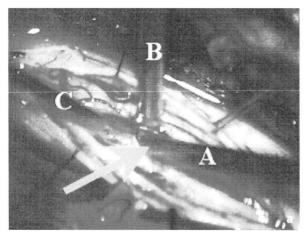

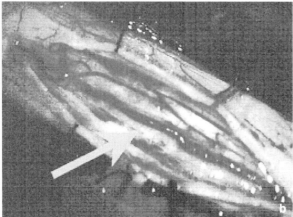

Fig. 1. (a) Punctate midline myelotomy with a 16 gauge needle (*A*) to a depth of 5 mm on either side of the median septum. Suction (*B*). The dorsal midline vein is gently mobilised (*C*). (b) Situs after the punctate midline myelotomy is performed (arrow) Reprint from R. Becker *et al.* Midline Myelotomy, Acta Neurochir (Wien) (1999) 141: 881–883 with permission

Discussion

The new technique of a punctate midline myelotomy, first described by Nauta *et al.*, obviously is not only effective in the treatment of visceral pain of hypogastric origin [5]. In the presented case an additional remarkable control of visceral pain of meso- and epigastric origin was observed. Meanwhile Nauta *et al.* reported on 5 additional patients, in whom PMM led to a sufficient pain reduction [6]. Kim and Kwon reported on sufficient control of visceral pain due to advanced stomach cancer after a modified Th 1–2 PMM [4].

While commissural midline myelotomies had been

performed with the intention to interrupt crossing fibres of the spinothalamic tract in the anterior white matter commissure, the limited approach of a punctate midline myelotomy to a depth of 5 mm is based on the anatomical concept of a dorsal midline visceral pain pathway [5].

Human surgical case studies with histological verification of the lesion and neuroanatomical and neurophysiological findings in animal experiments provided evidence that axons in the medial part of the posterior column at Th 10 convey ascending nociceptive signals from pelvic visceral organs. These visceral nociceptive afferents project to the ventral posterolateral nucleus of the thalamus via the nucleus gracilis. A restricted lesion in this area eliminated pelvic cancer pain without producing neurological deficits [1, 3].

As it was demonstrated, the punctate midline myelotomy (PMM) is obviously targeting a dorsal midline visceral pain pathway, that conveys not only pelvic nociceptive input but also nociceptive signals from the meso- and epigastrium [2, 4, 6]. When compared to the classical commissural midline myelotomy the technique described bears the advantage of a limited extension of a punctate lesion, which minimizes the risk of complications, which is of special importance in patients without neurological deficits.

References

1. Al-Chaer ED, Lawand NB, Westlund KN, Willis WD (1996) Visceral nociceptive input into the ventral posterolateral nucleus of the thalamus: a new function for the dorsal column pathway. J Neurophysiol 76(4): 2661–2674
2. Becker R, Sure U, Bertalanffy H (1999) Punctate midline myelotomy: a new approach in the management of visceral pain. Acta Neurochir (Wien) 141: 881–883
3. Hirshberg RM, Al-Chaer ED, Lawand NB, Westlund KN, Willis WD (1996) Is there a pathway in the posterior funiculus that signals visceral pain? Pain 67(2–3): 291–305
4. Kim YS, Kwon SJ (2000) High thoracic midline dorsal column myelotomy for severe visceral pain due to advanced stomach cancer. Neurosurgery 46(1): 85–90
5. Nauta HJ, Hewitt E, Westlund KN, Willis WD Jr (1997) Surgical interruption of a midline dorsal column visceral pain pathway. Case report and review of the literature. J Neurosurg 86(3): 538–542
6. Nauta HJ, Soukup VM, Fabian RH *et al* (2000) Punctate midline myelotomy for the relief of visceral cancer pain. J Neurosurg 92 [Suppl] 2: 125–130

Correspondence: Ralf Becker, M.D., Department of Neurosurgery, Philipps-University Hospital, Baldingerstraße, D-35033 Marburg, Germany.

Acta Neurochir (2001) [Suppl] 79: 79–82
© Springer-Verlag 2001

Deep Brain Stimulation Therapy for a Persistent Vegetative State

T. Yamamoto, Y. Katayama, H. Oshima, C. Fukaya, T. Kawamata, and **T. Tsubokawa**

Department of Neurological Surgery, Nihon University School of Medicine, Tokyo, Japan

Summary

Twenty cases of a persistent vegetative state (PVS) caused by various kinds of brain damage were neurologically and electrophysiologically evaluated at 3 months after persistence of the PVS, and were treated by deep brain stimulation (DBS) therapy. The stimulation sites were the mesencephalic reticular formation (2 cases) and CM-pf complex (18 cases). Seven of the patients emerged from the PVS, and became able to obey verbal commands. However, they remained in a bedridden state. These 7 cases revealed a desynchronization or slight desynchronization pattern on continuous EEG frequency analysis. The Vth wave of ABR and N20 of SEP could be recorded even with a prolonged latency, and the pain-related P250 was recorded with an amplitude of over 7 μV. We conclude that chronic DBS therapy may be useful for allowing the patient to emerge from a PVS, if the candidates are selected according to the neurophysiological criteria. In view of the severely disabled state of the patients who emerged from the PVS, a special rehabilitation program which includes neurostimulation therapy may be necessary for treatment of the PVS.

Keywords: Deep brain stimulation; vegetative state; CM-pf complex; EEG; evoked potential.

Introduction

As a result of progress in emergency treatment, many patients who would have died previously now recover. Although many lives are saved, the number of patients in a persistent vegetative state (PVS) is increasing. The PVS is a clinical condition involving complete unawareness of the self and environment, accompanied by sleep-wake cycles [3]. However, there are various grades of severity and various stages leading to various outcomes, even if the patient displays neurological signs identical to the PVS [5, 9, 10].

We evaluated patients in a PVS by an electrophysiological approach, and compared the results of the examinations with the long-term prognosis. As a result, we found that, even if the symptoms are similar from a neurological point of view, the degree of brain injury varies to a considerable degree. Also, there should be a large number of patients who may not be able to recover spontaneously, but who can be saved from the PVS by means of appropriate treatment.

In this paper, we report the long-term follow-up results of deep brain stimulation (DBS) therapy in comparison with the findings of electrophysiological evaluations in PVS patients.

Methods

Twenty patients in a PVS, who fell under the criteria of the Multi-Society Task Force on PVS (1994) [7, 8], were consecutively treated by chronic DBS therapy. All of these cases had been in a PVS for at least 3 months before the DBS therapy, and could be followed up for more than 2 years after the DBS therapy. Their ages ranged from 19 to 75 years old. The causes of the initial coma were head injury (9 cases), cerebrovascular accident (8 cases) and anoxia (3 cases). At 3 months after the onset of the comatose state, neurological examinations and neurophysiological evaluations were carried out. The neurophysiological evaluations included continuous EEG frequency analysis [9, 10] and assessments of the auditory brainstem response (ABR), somatosensory evoked potential (SEP) and pain-related P250 [4, 5].

We classified the continuous EEG frequency analysis into three types: (1) no desynchronization pattern: changes of peak frequency were present only in the alpha- and lower-frequencies, and not in the higher-frequencies; (2) slight desynchronization pattern: desynchronization was present but did not appear frequently; the duration was short, being under 10% of the time course, and the power of the high-frequency was low; and (3) desynchronization pattern: desynchronization (a change to low-amplitude and high-frequency) appeared frequently, and the increase in the high-frequency power was obvious at desynchronization. The ABR recordings were classified into three patterns: (1) no response; (2) prolonged latency of the Vth wave; and (3) normal recordings. Prolonged latency of the Vth wave meant that the I-V wave latency was over 2SD longer than in normal cases. The SEP recordings, on the well-preserved side in cases where laterality was present, were classified into three patterns: (1) no N20; (2) prolonged N20; and (3) normal N20. Prolonged latency of N20 meant that the Erb-N20 latency was over 2SD longer than in normal cases. The pain-related P250 recordings were classified into three patterns:

Table 1. *Neurological Grading Score of Persistent Vegetative State (Nihon University). A Grading is Obtained by Summing the Positive Items. The Score Ranges from 0 to 10 Points*

1	Alive with spontaneous respiration
2	Withdrawal response to pain
3	Spontaneous eye opening and closing
4	Spontaneous movement of extremities
5	Pursuit by eye movement
6	Emotional expression
7	Oral intake
8	Producing sound
9	Obeying orders
10	Verbal response

(1) no P250; (2) P250 recorded with under 7 µV; and (3) P250 recorded with over 7 µV.

The chronic DBS was applied using a chronically implanted flexible electrode under local anesthesia. As target points for the chronic DBS, the mesencephalic reticular formation (2 cases) and the CM-pf complex (18 cases) were selected. The stimulation was given every 2 to 3 hours during the daytime, and was continued for 30 min at one session. The frequency of the stimulation was mostly fixed at 25 Hz, and the intensity was decided according to the responses of each patient, being set at slightly higher than the threshold for inducing an arousal response.

To apply the chronic DBS, we employed a chronically implanted flexible electrode (3387, Medtronic Co.) and a transmitter-receiver system (3470 and 3425, Medtronic Co.). The target point in the mesencephalic reticular formation was the nucleus cuneiformis, which is located in the dorsal part of the nucleus ruber and ventral part of the deep layer of the superior colliculus. The CM-pf complex (P, 7–9; L, 5–6; H, 0–1) was selected as the stimulating point in the non-specific thalamic nucleus.

The follow-up results were evaluated every month after the operation employing the Neurological Grading Score of PVS (Table 1).

Results

Long-Term Follow-up Results

Within 12 months after the start of DBS therapy, 7 cases emerged from the PVS, and could communicate with some speech or responses, but needed some assistance for their everyday life in bed. Even after long-term rehabilitation, their state of being bedridden did not change. The other 13 cases could not communicate at all and failed to emerge from the PVS.

The main feature of the present stimulation therapy was that the patients presented strong arousal responses which were observed immediately at the start of stimulation. These strong arousal responses were seen in all 20 cases and had no relation to emergence or non-emergence from the PVS. At least 5 months of DBS therapy was necessary in order to emerge from

the PVS, and a rise in the Neurological Grading Score of PVS was observed within 3 months after commencement of the DBS therapy in effective cases.

As regards the cause of the initial coma, the effective cases had suffered brain damage through head injury or cerebrovascular accident, while the 3 cases of anoxia caused by cardiac arrest were among the non-effective cases.

Electrophysiological Classification

In the 7 cases that emerged from the PVS following DBS therapy, the Vth wave in ABR and N20 in SEP were recorded even with a longer-latency, the continuous EEG frequency analysis revealed a desynchronization pattern or slight desynchronization pattern, and the pain-related P250 was recorded with over 7 µV (Table 2).

Discussion

It is concluded that DBS can be effective for achieving emergence from the PVS, and an assessment of the possibility of recovery can be made before application of the treatment by checking the patient's neurological status and undertaking electrophysiological evaluations at 3 months after the initial insult. Patients whose electrophysiological evaluations revealed that a Vth wave in ABR and N20 in SEP were recordable even with a prolonged latency, a desynchronization pattern was noted on continuous EEG frequency analysis, and a pain-related P250 was recordable with over 7 µV, all emerged from the PVS. We consider therefore that electrophysiological evaluations are very important for assessing the resting neurological function in the PVS and for selecting candidates to undergo DBS therapy. We chose the given electrophysiological evaluations, because the ABR represents the function of the brainstem, SEP represents the function of the thalamocortical tract, continuous EEG frequency analysis represents the functional relationship between the brainstem and cerebral cortex, and pain-related P250 represents higher brain functions.

As reported previously, mesencephalic reticular formation and CM-pf complex stimulation elicits a strong arousal response and marked increases in r-CBF and r-CMRO$_2$ [10]. Electrical stimulation of the mesencephalic reticular formation induces EEG desynchronization; however, electrical stimulation of the CM-pf complex induces incremental recruiting and an aug-

Table 2. *Correlation Between Follow up Results of Chronic Deep Brain Stimulation and the Results of Electrophysiological Evaluations and Neurological Grading Score*

Case	Age sex (years)	Cause of coma	ABR	SEP	EEG	Pain-related P250	PVS before	Scale-after
1	58 F	vascular	prolonged V	prolonged N20	desynchronization	positive (over 7 uV)	5	10
2	75 M	trauma	prolonged V	prolonged N20	desynchronization	positive (over 7 uV)	4	9
3	43 M	vascular	prolonged V	prolonged N20	desynchronization	positive (over 7 uV)	4	9
4	19 F	vascular	prolonged V	prolonged N20	desynchronization	positive (over 7 uV)	5	9
5	59 F	vascular	prolonged V	prolonged N20	desynchronization	positive (over 7 uV)	3	9
6	41 F	vascular	prolonged V	prolonged N20	slight Desynchron.	positive (over 7 uV)	2	8
7	30 M	trauma	prolonged V	prolonged N20	slight Desynchron.	positive (over 7 uV)	5	8
8	56 M	trauma	prolonged V	prolonged N20	slight Desynchron.	positive (over 7 uV)	3	7
9	24 M	trauma	prolonged V	prolonged N20	no Desynchron.	positive (under 7 uV)	4	7
10	30 F	anoxia	prolonged V	prolonged N20	slight Desynchron.	positive (under 7 uV)	4	6
11	49 M	trauma	prolonged V	prolonged N20	slight Desynchron.	positive (over 7 uV)	3	6
12	29 M	trauma	prolonged V	prolonged N20	slight Desynchron.	positive (under 7 uV)	4	5
13	42 M	trauma	prolonged V	prolonged N20	slight Desynchron.	positive (under 7 uV)	3	5
14	44 M	anoxia	prolonged V	prolonged N20	no Desynchron.	positive (under 7 uV)	3	5
15	41 F	anoxia	prolonged V	no N20	no Desynchron.	positive (under 7 uV)	4	5
16	39 F	vascular	prolonged V	prolonged N20	no Desynchron.	positive (under 7 uV)	2	4
17	44 F	trauma	prolonged V	prolonged N20	no Desynchron.	positive (under 7 uV)	3	4
18	48 M	trauma	prolonged V	no N20	no Desynchron.	positive (under 7 uV)	2	3
19	61 F	vascular	prolonged V	no N20	no Desynchron.	negative	2	3
20	74 F	vascular	prolonged V	no N20	no Desynchron.	negative	2	3

ABR Auditory brainstem response, *SEP* somatosensory evoked potential, *EEG* continuous EEG frequency analysis, *PVS score* neurological grading score of PVS (before: at 3 months after brain injury, *after* after DBS and long term follow up results).

menting response on low-frequency stimulation, and EEG desynchronization on high-frequency stimulation [1, 2]. Luthi and McCormick [6] noted the importance of the low-threshold calcium spike and H-current in the waxing and waning of the EEG induced by CM-pf complex stimulation. We mainly selected the CM-pf complex as for the DBS therapy based on these two aspects of CM-pf complex stimulation. Since sleep-wake cycles accompany the PVS and thalamo-cortical function is more severely disturbed compared with that of the brainstem.

The Multi-Society Task Force on PVS (1994) [7, 8] listed the following as criteria for the vegetative state: 1) no evidence of awareness of self or environment and an inability to interact with others; 2) no evidence of sustained, reproducible, purposeful, or voluntary behavioral responses to visual, auditory, tactile, or noxious stimuli; 3) no evidence of language comprehension or expression; 4) intermittent wakefulness manifested by the presence of sleep-wake cycles; 5) sufficiently preserved hypothalamic and brainstem autonomic functions to permit survival with medical and nursing care; 6) bowel and bladder incontinence; and 7) variably preserved cranial-nerve reflexes (pupillary, oculocephalic, corneal, vestibulo-ocular, and gag) and

spinal reflexes. Further the Task Force defined the PVS as a vegetative state present at one month after brain injury. All of our cases matched the above criteria, and we wish to emphasize that all of our cases had remained in a PVS for at least 3 months before undergoing DBS therapy. We performed electrophysiological evaluations at 3 months after brain injury, and compared the findings with the long-term follow-up results. We observed some patients who showed recovery of their electrophysiological findings beyond 3 months. We wish therefore to emphasize the importance of the time schedule in undertaking electrophysiological evaluations for the purpose of predicting the prognosis.

It has been reported that recovery of consciousness from a posttraumatic PVS is unlikely after 12 months, and recovery from a nontraumatic PVS after 3 months is exceedingly rare [7, 8]. Our 7 cases who emerged from the PVS included 5 cases of cerebrovascular injury and 2 cases of traumatic injury. We concluded that chronic DBS therapy may be useful for allowing a patient to emerge from a PVS, if the candidates are selected according to the neurophysiological criteria. Our 7 cases, who emerged from the PVS and became able to obey verbal commands, continued in a bedridden state and could not live without some life support. In view of these results, we consider that a special rehabilitation program, which includes neurostimulation therapy and advanced rehabilitation for prolonged coma, may be necessary for treatment of the PVS.

References

1. Dempsey EWA, Morison RS (1942) A study of thalamo cortical relations. Am J Physiol 135: 291–292
2. Jasper HH, Naquet R, King LE (1955) Thalamocortical recruiting responses in sensory receiving areas in the cat. Electroencephalogr Clin Neurophysiol 7: 99–114
3. Jennett B, Plum F (1972) Persistent vegetative state after brain damage. Lancet 1: 734–737
4. Katayama Y, Tsubokawa T, Harano S, Tsukiyama T (1985) Dissociation of subjective pain report and pain-related late positive component of cerebral evoked potentials in subjects with brain lesions. Brain Res Bull 14: 423–426
5. Katayama Y, Tsubokawa T, Yamamoto T, Hirayama T, Miyazaki S, Koyoma S (1991) Characterization and modification of brain activity with deep brain stimulation in a persistent vegetative state. Pacing Clin Electrophysiol 14: 116–121
6. Luthi A, McCormick DA (1998) H-Current: Properties of a neuronal and network pacemaker. Neuron 21: 9–12
7. The Multi-Society Task Force on PVS (1994) Medical aspects of the persistent vegetative state (First of two parts). N Engl J Med 330: 1499–1508
8. The Multi-Society Task Force on PVS (1994) Medical aspects of the persistent vegetative state (Second of two parts). N Engl J Med 330: 1572–1579
9. Tsubokawa T, Yamamoto Y, Katayama Y, Hirayama T, Maejima S, Moriya T (1990) Deep brain stimulation in a persistent vegetative state: Follow-up results and criteria for selection of candidates. Brain Injury 4: 315–327
10. Tsubokawa T, Yamamoto T, Katayama Y (1990) Prediction of the outcome of prolonged coma caused by brain damage. Brain Injury 4: 329–337

Correspondence: Takamitsu Yamamoto, M.D., Ph.D., Department of Neurological Surgery, Nihon University School of Medicine, Tokyo 173, Japan.

Acta Neurochir (2001) [Suppl] 79: 83–88

Deep Brain Stimulation of the Globus Pallidus Internus (GPI) for Torsion Dystonia – A Report of two Cases

J. Vesper[1], **F. Klostermann**[2], **Th. Funk**[3], **F. Stockhammer**[1], and **M. Brock**[1]

[1] Department of Neurosurgery, University Medical Center Benjamin Franklin, Berlin, Germany
[2] Department of Neurology, University Medical Center Benjamin Franklin, Berlin, Germany
[3] Department of Neurosurgery, Klinikum Frankfurt, Frankfurt Oder, Germany

Summary

Generalized dystonia is known as a type of movement disorder in which pharmacotherapeutic options are very limited. Deep Brain Stimulation (DBS) is well established for Parkinson's disease (PD) and tremor dominant movement disorders. We report on two cases of generalized dystonia which were successfully treated by chronic high frequency stimulation in the Globus pallidus internus (GPI).

Two 26 and 27 years old males suffered from severe torsion dystonia and multisegmental dystonia of the lower limbs. Case 1 is a familiar type of dystonia (DYT1 positive). The onset of symptoms in both cases was at age 7. The complaints were initially treated with orally administered benzodiazepines, anticholinergic drugs, later by baclofen and L-DOPA. However there was no response. Case 2 was a patient with a history of left side dominated dystonia since the age of 8. It was first diagnosed as a psychogenic movement disorder. Prior to surgery he was treated with L-DOPA, anticholinergics, Baclofen without any effect. There was only a limited effect on high doses of diazepam. The patient is DYT1 negative.

The target point was on both sides the GPI. Intraoperative computerized tomography (CT) and ventriculography (VG) were used for target setting. Furthermore microrecordings were helpful to ensure the exact electrode position. Surgery was performed under analgosedation.

Two weeks after surgery we first observed a relief of symptoms in both cases. A significant reduction in the Burke-Fahn-Marsden-Dystonia Movement Rating Scale was observed at the 6 month follow-up (case 1: 95%, case 2: 80%). In case 1 a slight dystonic movement of the left ankle was the only remaining symptom under stimulation. The medication was continuously reduced. At the 24 month follow-up the effect of stimulation remained unchanged. However high stimualtion parameters are required to maintain an optimal effect (mean 3,5 V, 400 μs, 145 Hz).

Keywords: Dystonia; deep brain stimulation; stereotaxy; globus pallidus internus.

Introduction

Generalized dystonia is a severe form of movement disorder in which pharmacotherapeutic options are very limited. Dystonia was first described by Oppenheim. Since this time the disease is called dystonia musculorum deformans [10]. The basis of this disorder is a deterioration of basal ganglia control mechanisms, particulary the striatal control of the pallidum and the pars reticulata of the substantia nigra [10, 11]. Recently SPECT (Single-Photon-Emission-Computerized-Tomography) studies proved also a dysfunction of the dopaminergic system [11]. Dystonia may occur after severe head injury. In these cases a kinetic tremor is often observed [10]. Fahn *et al.* developed a classification system of dystonia in order to explain the changes in the basal ganglia circuit [10]. Genetic alterations are also responsible for dystonia, especially in hereditary cases [22]. The DYT-1-gene is a typical finding in these patients with primary dystonia.

Classification of dystonia is performed according to the reason of onset in primary and secondary dystonias. Secondary dystonias are often due to hypoxia. Treatment of those cases is more difficult due to the additional complaints of these patients [10].

Pharmacotherapy is limited, however some improvement has been reported under treatment with L-DOPA, Baclofen, anticholinergics and benzodiazepine. Particulary in cases of generalized torsion dystonia pharmacotherapy is usually unsuccessful [9].

For 20 years these patients were treated also with pallidotomy. Since this method has a high rate of permanent morbidity, conservative treatment was preferred [23]. Until now surgery for dystonic patients was limited to spinal cord stimulation and drug administration devices.

Deep Brain Stimulation is well established for Parkinson's disease and tremordominant movement disorders. It has induced a renaissance of stereotactic surgery for movement disorders [14, 31, 32]. The accuracy of this method was also influenced by both a deeper understanding of the pathophysiologic relations in the basal ganglia and an optimization of imaging techniques. Furthermore deep brain microrecordings enable an additional intraoperative target control [24, 37]. Pharmacoresistant cases of Parkinson's disease and tremor dominant disorders are classical indications for stererotactic surgery.

Two cases are reported with severe generalized and multisegmental types of dystonia. They were successfully treated by chronic high frequency stimulation.

Case Reports

Case 1

An at the time of surgery 26 year old male had suffered from symptoms of dystonia since the age of 7. Starting with dystonia of the left foot, he very fast developed severe dystonia of the lower limbs. This was first treated with benzodiazepines, later with baclofen p.o.. The patient was severly handicaped (Burke-Fahn-Marsden-Dystonia-Rating-Scale, movement: 57, 5 points, disability: 16 points, Figs: 2 and 3) [3]. The genetic evaluation revealed a DYT1 positive status. A sister of his mother suffered from similar symptoms, however less severe. Because of the rapid progression of the disease a cervical spinal cord stimulator was implanted with a transient success. After a mild trauma of the spine a dislocation of the electrode was diagnosed, which could not have been resolved whith surgical revision. Due to the fact of further progression of the disease the patient became wheelchair bound and resistant to oral medication. An implanted pump revealed limited success in administrating baclofen intrathecally. Finally the patient was treated with 980 μg/d Baclofen intrathecally and up to 100 mg/d diazepam. Under these conditions the patient remained wheelchair bound with severe lower limb dystonia.

Case 2

A 27 year old male suffered from signs of generalized dystonia since the age of 8 years. It started with symptoms in the neck and torsions of the left arm. Patient developed severe gait disturbances and a thoracic spine scoliosis due to the progression of dystonia (BFMDRS movement: 48 points, disability: 11 points, Figs: 2 and 3), [3]. Initially he was treated with antipsychotic medication without success. After several weeks in a psychiatric clinic any medication failed to reduce the progression of the torsion. Finally the diagnosis of a psychogenic movement disorder was established and the patient was discharged. For more than 10 years no medical treatment was applied. During the stage in our outpatient department anticholinergics, baclofen and L-DOPA were administered. However none of these medication was successful. Only a limited improvement was seen after high dose diazepam.

Material and Methods

Surgery was performed under analgosedation. Target calculation was performed using computerized tomography and ventriculography. The Leibinger system according to Riechert and Mundinger was used in all cases. Coordinates of the internal pallidum were calculated by means of the Schaltenbrand-Wahren atlas [33]. Surgery started on the left brain side. Previously calculated target points were transferred to the target simulator. Spontaneous discharges were recorded using a semi-microrecording electrode, starting 20 mm above the target area. The border between external and internal pallidum was determined in this way. Visual evoked potentials were recorded in order to determine the proximity to the optic tract. X-ray images were performed for determination of final electrode coordinates. Final electrode (Medtronic 3387) was implanted under fluoroscopic control. In case 1 we used ITREL® II (Medtronic Inc., Minneapolis, MN, USA) neurostimulation system bilaterally. Case 2 had received a dual-channel KINETRA™ system (Medtronic Inc., Minneapolis, MN, USA) which allows bilateral electrode control. (Fig. 1). There were neither surgical nor general complications in both patients.

Patients were evaluated preoperatively and 1 week postoperatively as well as 3, 6 and 12 months postoperatively. This was performed using the Burke-Fahn-Marsden-Dystonia Rating Scale (BFMDRS) [3].

Statistic evaluation included multivariance analysis with the one way ANOVA-rank-sum test (Sigmastat, Jandel Scientific Inc, Chicago, IL, USA).

Results

Case 1

After two weeks a first improvement was observed. The patient was able to stand with assistance. At the three month follow-up the patient walked without assistance. Slight dystonic movement of the left ankle was the only remaining symptom under stimulation. This was additionally treated with an orthopedic tool.

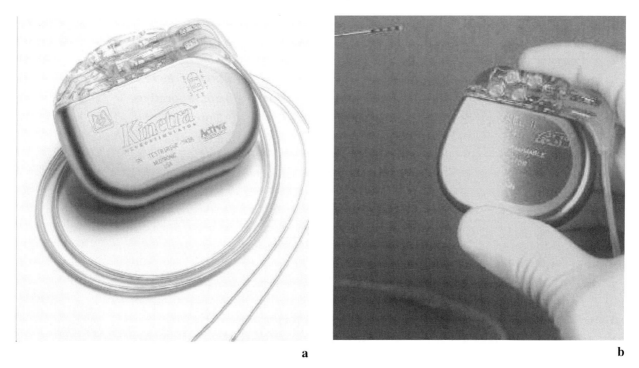

a   b

Fig. 1. KINETRA and ITREL

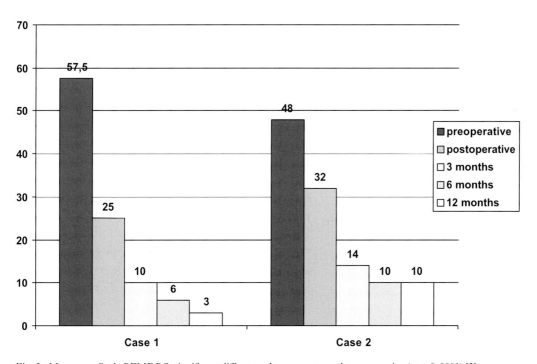

Fig. 2. Movement Scale BFMDRS, significant differences between pre- and postoperative (p < 0, 0001) [3]

The oral medication was reduced. After 6 months it was stopped. Then the intrathecal baclofen was reduced continuously. In case 2 patient torsions have markedly been reduced by means of DBS. The patient is now able to perform all activities of daily living. A significant reduction (95%) in the BFMDRS was established (Figs. 2 and 3). High stimulation parameters are nessessary to maintain the effect (Table 1) (left:

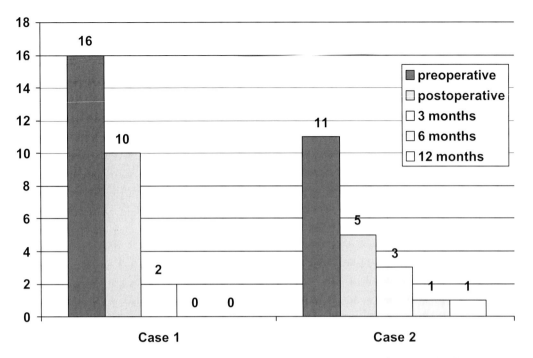

Fig. 3. Disability Scale BFMDRS, significant differences between pre- and postoperative (p < 0,0001) [3]

Table 1. *Stimulation Parameters 6 Months Postoperatively*

	Case 1		Case 2	
	Left	Right	Left	Right
Amplitude (V)	3,6	3,6	4,0	2,0
Frequency (Hz)	160	160	132	132
Pulse Width (μs)	450	400	210	150
Impedance (Ω)	971	1035	1015	1020
Output (μA)	248	214	132	85

3,6 V, 400 µs, 135 Hz, right: 2,5 V, 450 µs, 160 Hz). After 24 months the effect of DBS was unchanged. The patient remained physically independent.

Case 2

Initial stimulation parameters were high in order to obtain a maximal functional lesion in the target area (3,5 V, 180 µs, 135 Hz) (Table 1). Improvement of dystonic symptoms was observed after 3 days in the left arm. This remained stable during the following weeks. After 6 months a significant and ongoing improvement was established (Figs. 2 and 3). The patient became able to finish his professional education. He is still under physiotherapy due to his severe scoliosis. The oral medication is continued with 15 mg dia-

zepam daily. However high stimulation parameters are required on the left side, too. (Table 1).

Discussion

Generalized torsion dystonia is an extrapyramidal movement disorder with limited options for pharmacotherapy. Benzodiazepines, Baclofen, L-DOPA and Botulinum toxin are the most important groups of medication [9]. Because of the limited effect of pharmacotherapy, particulary in generalized types of dystonia, several surgical attempts were started in order to improve the motor symptoms of this disease. Until now, surgical skill was to produce a lesion to interrupt the disturbed pathways. Therefore pallidotomy was mainly performed. The success is limited due to the risk of severe permanent additional neurological deficits. Particulary hemiballisms may occur as in pallidotomy for Parkinson's disease. [1, 2, 4, 8, 12, 15, 18, 22, 23, 24, 27, 28, 36, 39, 40, 42]. Furthermore pallidotomy may lead to deteriorations of the optic tract. [1, 5, 13, 23].

However in series with a small number of patients a long-term effectiveness has been reported recently [16, 29, 30].

By means of deep brain stimulation (DBS) of the globus pallidum internum (GPI) an alternative surgical treatment was developed for extrapyramidal movement disorders. It offers a method with less side effects and low surgical risks. There is no permanent lesion of brain tissue. Side effects can be avoided by changing stimulation parameters. This method was primarily applied in patients with tremor dominant disorders, later also in akinetic–rigid parkinsonian conditions. Initial target points were found in the GPI and for tremor dominant disorders into the ventral intermediate thalamic nucleus (VIM). Later subthalamic nucleus (STN) was determined as the optimal target [25].

Based on the high efficacy of DBS for tremor and akinetic symptoms dystonia came up to be also treated in this way. Dystonia is also a secondary symptom in Parkinson's disease. It has markedly been reduced in patients with GPI stimulation. Until now there are only few preliminary reports [6, 20, 21, 38]. Targets were determined according to the experiences of pallidotomy and to the coordinates of the Schaltenbrand-Wahren atlas [7, 12, 17, 19, 29, 31, 34, 35, 36, 40, 42, 43].

Single-unit microrecordings from the different structures of the basal ganglia along the trajectory are useful to have an electrophysiologic target confirmation. Visual evoked potentials revealed a determination of the proximity to the optical tract [18, 23, 26, 27, 37, 41, 43].

Postoperative setting of the stimulation parameters was performed in order to achieve an optimal effect without stimulation dependent side effects. Compared to parameters for Parkinson's disease and tremor high output values were required in both patients. An explanation for this observation is the larger anatomic dimension and the heterogeneous structure of the GPI compared to the STN. More energy is required to achieve a similar functional lesion effect in the GPI. The battery survival is therefore limited to approximately 24 months. Replacement can be performed with a small procedure under local anaesthesia.

A drastic reduction of dystonic symptoms was achieved in both patients (Figs. 2 and 3). It was maintained over the follow-up course of 12 months. After electrode placement a continuous improvement was observed until the 6 month follow-up examination. The reason for this delayed effect remains undetected. Further investigations using functional imaging are required to determine the potential influence of brain plasticity.

Cases 1 and 2 were patients with primary dystonia. Whether or not secondary (e.g. due to perinatal hypo-

xia) dystonias are also candidates for surgery is still under controversial discussion.

Conclusion

Chronic high frequency stimulation of the Globus pallidus internus is long-term effective in severe types of generalized and multisegmental dystonia. It improves both the motoric symptoms and the quality of life. The different side effects of lesional procedures can be avoided.

Further investigations with larger patient groups are required in order to confirm these preliminary results by prospective and randomized trials. The options for secondary dystonias are still undefined.

References

1. Bertrand C, Molina-Negro P, Martinez SN (1978) Combined stereotactic and peripheral surgical approach for spasmodic torticollis. Appl Neurophysiol 41(1–4): 122–133
2. Bhatia KP, Marsden CD, Thomas DG (1998) Posteroventral pallidotomy can ameliorate attacks of paroxysmal dystonia induced by exercise [letter]. J Neurol Neurosurg Psychiatry 65(4): 604–605
3. Burke RE, Fahn S, Marsden CD, Bressmann SB, Friedman J (1985) Validity and reliability of rating scale for primary torsion dystonias. Neurol 35: 73–77
4. Cardoso F, Jankovic J, Grossman RG, Hamilton WJ (1995) Outcome after stereotactic thalamotomy for dystonia and hemiballismus. Neurosurgery 36(3): 501–508
5. Cohn MC, Hudgins PA, Sheppard SK, Starr PA, Bakay RA (1998) Pre- and postoperative MR evaluation of stereotactic pallidotomy. AJNR Am J Neuroradiol 19(6): 1075–1080
6. Coubes P, Echenne B, Roubertie A, Vayssiere N, Tuffery S, Humbertclaude V et al (1999) [Treatment of early-onset generalized dystonia by chronic bilateral stimulation of the internal globus pallidus. Apropos of a case]. Neurochirurgie 45(2): 139–144
7. Dalvi A, Winfield L, Yu Q, Cote L, Goodman RR, Pullman SL (1999) Stereotactic posteroventral pallidotomy: clinical methods and results at 1-year follow-up. Mov Disord 14(2): 256–261
8. de Bie RM, Schuurman PR, de Haan PS, Bosch DA, Speelman JD (1999) Unilateral pallidotomy in advanced Parkinson's disease: a retrospective study of 26 patients. Mov Disord 14(6): 951–957
9. Durif F (1999) Treating and preventing levodopa-induced dyskinesias: current and future strategies. Drugs Aging 14(5): 337–345
10. Fahn S, Bressman SB, Marsden CD (1998) Classification of dystonia. Adv Neurol 78: 1–10
11. Fahn S (1988) Concept and classification of dystonia. Adv Neurol 50: 1–8
12. Favre J, Taha JM, Nguyen TT, Gildenberg PL, Burchiel KJ (1996) Pallidotomy: a survey of current practice in North America. Neurosurgery 39(4): 883–890
13. Friedman DP, Goldman HW, Flanders AE (1997) MR imaging of stereotaxic pallidotomy and thalamotomy. AJR Am J Roentgenol 169(3): 894–896

14. Grossman RG (1988) Surgery for movement disorders. Parkinson's disease and movement disorders. In: Jankovic JJ, Tolosa E (eds) Urban and Schwarzenberg, Baltimore Munich, pp 461–469

15. Hariz MI, Hirabayashi H (1997) Is there a relationship between size and site of the stereotactic lesion and symptomatic results of pallidotomy and thalamotomy? Stereotact Funct Neurosurg 69(1–4 Pt 2): 28–45

16. Iacono RP, Kuniyoshi SM, Lonser RR, Maeda G, Inae AM, Ashwal S (1996) Simultaneous bilateral pallidoansotomy for idiopathic dystonia musculorum deformans. Pediatr Neurol 14(2): 145–148

17. Iacono RP, Shima F, Lonser RR, Kuniyoshi S, Maeda G, Yamada S (1995) The results, indications, and physiology of posteroventral pallidotomy for patients with Parkinson's disease [see comments]. Neurosurgery 36(6): 1118–1125

18. Justesen CR, Penn RD, Kroin JS, Egel RT (1999) Stereotactic pallidotomy in a child with Hallervorden-Spatz disease. Case report. J Neurosurg 90(3): 551–554

19. Kopyov O, Jacques D, Duma C, Buckwalter G, Kopyov A, Lieberman A *et al* (1997) Microelectrode-guided posteroventral medial radiofrequency pallidotomy for Parkinson's disease. J Neurosurg 87(1): 52–59

20. Krauss JK, Pohle T, Weber S, Ozdoba C, Burgunder JM (1999) Bilateral stimulation of globus pallidus internus for treatment of cervical dystonia. Lancet 354(9181): 837–838

21. Kumar R, Dagher A, Hutchinson WD, Lang AE, Lozano AM (1999) Globus pallidus deep brain stimulation for generalized dystonia, clinical and PET investigation. Neurology 53(4): 871–874

22. Lai T, Lai JM, Grossman RG (1999) Functional recovery after bilateral pallidotomy for the treatment of early-onset primary generalized dystonia. Arch Phys Med Rehabil 80(10): 1340–1342

23. Laitinen LV, Bergenheim AT, Hariz MI (1992) Ventroposterolateral pallidotomy can abolish all parkinsonian symptoms. Stereotact Funct Neurosurg 58(1–4): 14–21

24. Lenz FA, Suarez JI, Metman LV, Reich SG, Karp BI, Hallett M *et al* (1998) Pallidal activity during dystonia: somatosensory reorganisation and changes with severity. J Neurol Neurosurg Psychiatry 65(5): 767–770

25. Limousin-Dowsey P, Pollak P, Van Blercom N, Krack P, Benazzouz A, Benabid A (1999) Thalamic, subthalamic nucleus and internal pallidum stimulation in Parkinson's. J Neurol 246 [Suppl] 2: II42–II45

26. Lin JJ, Lin GY, Shih C, Lin SZ, Chang DC, Lee CC (1999) Benefit of bilateral pallidotomy in the treament of generalized dystonia. Case report. J Neurosurg 90(5): 974–976

27. Lin JJ, Lin SZ, Chang DC (1999) Pallidotomy and generalized dystonia [letter]. Mov Disord 14(6): 1057–1059

28. Lin JJ, Lin SZ, Lin GY, Chang DC, Lee CC (1998) Application of bilateral sequential pallidotomy to treat a patient with generalized dystonia. Eur Neurol 40(2): 108–110

29. Lozano AM, Kumar R, Gross RE, Giladi N, Hutchison WD, Dostrovsky JO *et al* (1997) Globus pallidus internus pallidotomy for generalized dystonia. Mov Disord 12(6): 865–870

30. Ondo WG, Desaloms JM, Jankovic J, Grossman RG (1998) Pallidotomy for generalized dystonia. Mov Disord 13(4): 693–698

31. Ostertag CB, Lucking CH, Mehdorn HM, Deuschl G (1997) [Stereotactic treatment of movement disorders]. Nervenarzt 68(6): 477–484

32. Poewe W (1999) What is new in movement disorders? Wien Klin Wochenschr 111(17): 664–671

33. Schaltenbrand G, Wahren W (1977) Atlas for stereotaxy of the human brain. Thieme, Stuttgart

34. Schuurman PR, de Bie RM, Speelman JD, Bosch DA (1997) Bilateral posteroventral pallidotomy in advanced Parkinson's disease in three patients. Mov Disord 12(5): 752–755

35. Schuurman PR, de Bie RM, Speelman JD, Bosch DA (1997) Posteroventral pallidotomy in movement disorders. Acta Neurochir (Wien) [Suppl] 68: 14–17

36. Sutton JP, Couldwell W, Lew MF, Mallory L, Grafton S, DeGiorgio C *et al* (1995) Ventroposterior medial pallidotomy in patients with advanced Parkinson's disease. Neurosurgery 36(6): 1112–1116

37. Tan AK, Yeo TT, Tijia HAT, Khanna S, Nowinski WL (1998) Stereotactic microelectrode-guided posteroventral pallidotomy and pallidal deep brain stimulation for Parkinon's disease. Ann Acad Med Singapore 27(6): 767–771

38. Tronnier VM, Fogel W (2000) Pallidal stimulation for generalized dystonia. Report of three cases. J Neurosurg 92(3): 453–456

39. Tsubokawa T, Katayama Y, Yamamoto T (1995) Control of persistent hemiballismus by chronic thalamic stimulation. J Neurosurg 82: 501–505

40. Vitek JL, Bakay RA (1997) The role of pallidotomy in Parkinson's disease and dystonia. Curr Opin Neurol 10(4): 332–339

41. Vitek JL, Chockkan V, Zhang JY, Kaneoke Y, Evatt M, DeLong MR *et al* (1999) Neuronal activity in the basal ganglia in patients with generalized dystonia and hemiballismus. Ann Neurol 46(1): 22–35

42. Vitek JL, Zhang J, Evatt M, Mewes K, DeLong MR, Hashimoto T, Triche S, Bakay RA (1998) Gpi pallidotomy for dystonia: clinical outcome and neuronal activity. Adv Neurol 78: 211–219

43. Weetman J, Anderson IM, Gregory RP, Gill SS (1997) Bilateral posteroventral pallidotomy for severe antipsychotic induced tardive dyskinesia and dystonia [letter]. J Neurol Neurosurg Psychiatry 63(4): 554–556

Correspondence: Dr. J. Vesper, Department of Neurosurgery, University Medical Center Benjamin Franklin, Berlin, Germany.

Acta Neurochir (2001) [Suppl] 79: 89–92

Control of Post-Stroke Movement Disorders Using Chronic Motor Cortex Stimulation

Y. Katayama, H. Oshima, C. Fukaya, T. Kawamata, and **T. Yamamaoto**

Department of Neurological Surgery, Nihon University School of Medicine, Tokyo, Japan

Summary

The effects of motor cortex (MC) stimulation on post-stroke movement disorders were analyzed in 50 patients. These individuals either underwent MC stimulation primarily for the purpose of controlling their post-stroke involuntary movements (n = 8) or underwent MC stimulation for the purpose of controlling their post-stroke central pain (n = 42). In the latter patients, the effects of MC stimulation on co-existent involuntary or voluntary movement disorders were analyzed retrospectively. Good control of involuntary movements was observed in 2 of 3 patients with hemichoreo-athetosis, 2 of 2 patients with distal resting or action tremor, and 1 of 3 patients with proximal postural tremor. Subjective improvements in motor performance were reported by 8 patients who had mild motor weakness, and the effects appeared to be attributable to attenuation of rigidity. We consider that these findings justify further clinical studies on MC stimulation for the control of post-stroke movement disorders.

Keywords: Involuntary movement; motor cortex; rigidity; stimulation; stroke; tremor.

Introduction

Movement disorders are one of the most disabling sequelae of stroke. During the last decade, it has become clear that chronic stimulation of certain brain areas produces a dramatic improvement in the symptoms of movement disorders [1, 2, 6, 8, 9]. Cooper et al. [4] reported that clinically useful improvement was noted after deep brain stimulation in 6 of 9 cases with unspecified involuntary movements caused by stroke. Andy [1] has also described a case in which thalamic syndrome with choreiform movements following stroke was successfully treated by deep brain stimulation. We have reported patients in whom stimulation of the contralateral thalamic nucleus ventralis intermedius (VIM) provided excellent control of persistent hemiballismus, hemichoreo-athetosis and distal resting or action tremors caused by stroke [6, 9].

We previously found that excellent pain control can sometimes be achieved in post-stroke central pain patients undergoing stimulation of the contralateral cortex [5]. The area providing strong pain inhibition appeared to correspond to the motor cortex (MC), since such an area caused muscle contraction if stimulated at a higher intensity. In the course of clinical trials on MC stimulation for controlling post-stroke central pain, we encountered some patients who were delighted by an unexpected improvement during such stimulation therapy in their involuntary or voluntary movement disorders caused by stroke [5–7, 9]. These observations suggest that MC stimulation may be potentially useful for the control of post-stroke movement disorders.

Materials and Methods

A total of 48 patients underwent MC stimulation, 6 patients primarily for the purpose of controlling post-stroke involuntary movements and the remaining 42 for the purpose of controlling their post-stroke central pain (Table 1). In the latter patients, the effects of MC stimulation on co-existent involuntary or voluntary movement disorders were analyzed retrospectively. Among the 48 patients, 8 demonstrated various types of involuntary movements: hemichorea-athetosis (rapid, flexion-extension, rotation or crossing movements of one side of the body with distal predominance) associated with thalamic infarct or hemorrhage in 3, distal resting and/or action tremor (a relatively fine oscillation of the distal segment of the limbs occurring at rest or on action) associated with multiple lacunar, striatal or thalamic infarcts in 2, and proximal postural tremor (a relatively coarse oscillation of the proximal segment of the limbs which tended to increase in amplitude with prolonged posture and to persist or worsen with goal-directed movements) associated with infarct or hemorrhage within the midbrain or thalamic regions in 3. The patients and their families gave informed consent for the procedures described below to be carried out. This study was approved by the Committee for Clinical Trials and Research on Humans.

The surgical methods employed in the present series of patients were basically similar to those reported by us previously [5, 7]. Briefly, MC stimulation was performed with an electrode array consisting of 4 plate electrodes (5 mm in diameter, each separated by 5 mm; Medtronic Inc., USA), which was put in place epidurally through a small craniotomy. In general, the location of the MC was determined from muscle contractions in response to bipolar stimulation with electrical pulses having a low frequency. When muscle contractions could not be observed, no matter how extensively we attempted to determine the appropriate stimulation sites, several electrode arrays were placed in parallel around the location of the MC which was estimated by somatosensory evoked potential and/or neuroimaging techniques. Anticonvulsants were administered to all patients throughout the therapy with MC stimulation.

The electrode leads were externalized for 4–7 days for test stimulation. During the test stimulation period, stimuli were delivered using various combinations of electrodes by employing pulses mostly with a duration of 0.1–0.5 ms. The intensity of MC stimulation was carefully restricted below the threshold for muscle contraction and the frequency was below 50 Hz, since we had been employing this range of frequency for MC stimulation in pain control. None of our patients subjected to MC stimulation developed either observable or electroencephalographic seizure activity spontaneously after internalization. When stimulation was applied at intensities above the threshold of muscle contraction at a higher frequency, short-lasting generalized seizures were induced in some patients only in association with the stimulation. If the patients were satisfied by the effect of the stimulation, the electrodes were internalized. Chronic stimulation was performed using an appropriate stimulation system (Medtronic Inc., USA). Stimulation was applied bipolarly with various combinations of electrodes by employing pulses mostly with a duration of 0.1–0.2 ms and other parameters which achieved the best effects in each individual patient. The follow-up periods after electrode implantation ranged from 2 to 7 years.

Results

Effects on Involuntary Movements

The effects of MC stimulation varied depending on the types of involuntary movements (Table 1). In 2 of the 3 patients with hemichoreo-athetosis, the involuntary movements were appreciably attenuated by the MC stimulation. However, the stimulation system was not internalized in these patients for the following reasons. In one patient, the purpose of MC stimulation was to control his co-existent post-stroke pain, and the actual effect of the MC stimulation for this purpose was not satisfactory. In the remaining 2 patients, VIM stimulation afforded better control of the involuntary movements, so that he underwent internalization of the stimulation system for VIM stimulation.

In both of the 2 patients who demonstrated distal resting and/or action tremor, the tremor was completely abolished by MC stimulation. In these patients, the stimulation system was internalized for the purpose of controlling co-existent post-stroke central pain. When the MC stimulation attenuated the involuntary movements, such an effect began to be observed immediately after the start of stimulation, and reappeared after termination of the stimulation. The effects on involuntary movements occurred at an intensity below the threshold for muscle contraction and a relatively high frequency of more than 75 Hz. However, we restricted the frequency to below 50 Hz, which is sufficient for pain control. The inhibition of tremor was partial in this frequency range. In contrast to the distal resting or action tremor, proximal postural tremor was not well controlled by MC stimulation: only one of the 3 patients demonstrated partial attenuation of her involuntary movements. She was not satisfied by such partial control, so that the stimulation system was not internalized.

Effects on Voluntary Movements

The 42 patients who underwent MC stimulation primarily for the purpose of controlling their post-stroke central pain, demonstrated varying degrees of motor weakness ranging from mild to severe. Muscle contraction was inducible in the painful area in 29 patients intraoperatively when the MC was stimulated at a higher intensity. No such muscle response was inducible in the remaining patients, even though extensive exploration was performed to determine the appropriate stimulation sites.

Subjective improvement of motor performance, which had been impaired in association with mild or moderate motor weakness, was reported by 8 patients during MC stimulation (Table 1). No improvement of motor performance was experienced in patients who

Table 1. *Effects of MC Stimulation on Post-Stroke Movement Disorders*

Symptoms	n	No. with beneficial effects	No. with internalization
Hemichorea-athetosis	3	2	0
Distal resting or action tremor	2	2	2
Proximal postural tremor	3	1	0
Motor weakness		8	8*
Total	48	13	10

* Excluding patients in whom the stimulation system was internalized for pain control without appreciable effects on motor performance.

demonstrated severe motor weakness and/or no muscle contraction in response to MC stimulation at a higher intensity. The improvement of motor performance occurred at an intensity below the threshold for muscle contraction and within the frequency range employed for pain control.

It was not evident objectively that muscle strength was elevated by MC stimulation. The improved motor performance appeared most probably to have resulted from attenuation of rigidity. Subjective improvements of motor performance were reported regardless of whether the pain was satisfactorily controlled by the MC stimulation or not. In one patient who experienced no pain control with MC stimulation, the stimulation system was, nevertheless, internalized because he was so pleased by the marked improvement that occurred in his motor performance.

Discussion

While the benefit afforded by ablative surgical treatments for post-stroke involuntary movements is unpredictable, the surgical lesions are irreversible and unalterable once they are produced. In post-stroke patients, ablative procedures applied to the damaged brain should be minimized. Stimulation therapy is a better option due to the reversibility of the procedure and the alterability of the anatomical location and extent of stimulation following surgery.

The results of the present study indicate that MC stimulation can bring about control of post-stroke involuntary movements, similarly to VIM stimulation [6, 9]. This finding is consistent with earlier investigations which demonstrated that MC stimulation can inhibit involuntary movements of other etiologies [3, 10]. For example, Woolsey et al. [10] showed that, in severe Parkinson's disease, marked inhibition of the tremor could be induced by MC stimulation. The MC is the last relay of complex extrapyramidal neuronal loops which finally join the pyramidal tract. It has long been recognized that post-stroke involuntary movements cannot occur unless the pyramidal tract is able to function. The effects of MC stimulation observed in the present study may be related to a desynchronization of abnormal activities which are transmitted from the extrapyramidal neuronal loops to the pyramidal tract. Post-stroke involuntary movements, especially those in thalamic syndrome, are sometimes associated with central pain. Stimulation of the VIM could elicit opposite effects in these disorders: involuntary movements can be attenuated, but the pain of the same patients may be exacerbated. The present results suggested that MC stimulation might represent the therapy of choice under such circumstances.

The effects of MC stimulation on tremor occurred at intensities below the threshold for muscle contraction and at a relatively high frequency. While the frequency employed for clinical use in the present study was limited to below 50 Hz, higher frequencies appear to afford better control of post-stroke movement disorders. Future studies to ascertain the safety of applying higher frequency stimulation could enhance the value of MC stimulation in controlling involuntary movements.

The present study also demonstrated that MC stimulation could improve the motor performance of patients with motor weakness. Such an effect appeared to be associated with an attenuated rigidity rather than an increased muscle strength. This inference is again consistent with earlier studies which revealed a marked inhibition of rigidity during MC stimulation [10]. Taken together, these observations imply that MC stimulation may be useful in many patients to control a variety of post-stroke movement disorders if an appropriate technique for MC stimulation can be established. We consider that the present findings justify further clinical studies on MC stimulation.

Acknowledgment

This work was supported by Grants-in-Aid for Scientific Research from the Ministry of Education, Science and Culture (B09470302 and A12307029), and a Program Grant from the Ministry of Health and Welfare (H11-Research on Specific Diseases-52), Japan.

References

1. Andy OJ (1983) Thalamic stimulation for control of movement disorders. Appl Neurophysiol 46: 107–111
2. Benabid AL, Pollack P, Louveau A, Henry S, de Rougemont J (1987) Combined (thalamotomy and stimulation) stereotactic surgery of the VIM thalamic nucleus for bilateral parkinson disease. Appl Neurophysiol 50: 344–346
3. Britton TC, Thompson PD, Day BL, Rothwell JC, Findley LJ, Marsden CD (1993) Modulation of postural wrist tremors by magnetic stimulation of the motor cortex in patients with Parkinson's disease or essential tremor and in normal subjects mimicking tremor. Ann Neurol 33: 473–479
4. Cooper IS, Upton ARM, Amin I (1982) Chronic cerebellar stimulation (CCS) and deep brain stimulation (DBS) in involuntary movement disorders. Appl Neurophysiol 45: 209–217
5. Katayama Y, Fukaya C, Yamamoto T (1998) Post-stroke pain control by chronic motor cortex stimulation. Neurological characteristics predicting a favorable response. J Neurosurg 78: 585–591

Acta Neurochir (2001) [Suppl] 79: 93–98
© Springer-Verlag 2001

Vagus Nerve Stimulation for Epilepsy, Clinical Efficacy of Programmed and Magnet Stimulation

P. Boon[1], K. Vonck[1], P. Van Walleghem[1], M. D'Havé[1], J. Caemaert[2], and J. De Reuck[1]

[1] Epilepsy Monitoring Unit, Department of Neurology, Ghent University Hospital, Belgium
[2] Department of Neurosurgery, Ghent University Hospital, Belgium

Summary

Rationale. Vagus nerve stimulation (VNS) by intermittent and programmed electrical stimulation of the left vagus nerve in the neck, has become widely available. It is an effective treatment for patients with refractory epilepsy. Patients can be provided with a magnet that allows to deliver additional stimulation trains. Since earlier studies have demonstrated the persistence of a stimulation effect after discontinuation of the stimulation train, we evaluated the clinical efficacy of VNS both in the programmed intermittent stimulation mode and magnet stimulation mode.

Methods. A group of 30 patients (16 F, 14 M) with medically refractory partial epilepsy, who were unsuitable candidates for resective surgery, were included in the study. The patients, their companions and caregivers were instructed on how to administer additional stimulation trains using a hand-held magnet when an aura or a seizure onset occurred. Patients or caregivers could recognize habitual seizures and were able to evaluate sudden interruption of these seizures. Using seizure diaries, detailed accounts of magnet use and regular clinic follow-up visits, data on seizure frequency and severity and number of magnet applications were collected. Patients who provided unreliable information were excluded from the analysis.

Results. Forty-seven percent of all patients had an improvement in seizure control with a reduction in seizure frequency of more than 50% during a mean follow-up of 33 months (range: 4–67 months). More than half of the patients used the magnet and provided reliable information. In 63% of patients who were able to self-administer or receive additional magnet stimulation, seizures could be interrupted, be it consistently or occasionally. More than half of the patients who reported a positive effect of magnet stimulation became responders. In most cases the magnet was applied by a caregiver.

Conclusions. To our knowledge, this study is the first to explore the efficacy of magnet-induced vagus nerve stimulation. Results suggest that the magnet is a useful tool that provides patients and mainly caregivers with an additional means of controlling refractory seizures. Additional controlled studies comparing programmed stimulation and magnet-induced stimulation in monitoring conditions are warranted.

Keywords: Epilepsy; vagus nerve stimulation; efficacy; magnet-induced stimulation.

Introduction

Electrical stimulation of the left vagus nerve is an adjunctive therapy for patients with refractory epilepsy who are unsuitable candidates for resective or disconnective epilepsy surgery or who have had insufficient benefit from such treatments. The effect of vagus nerve stimulation both on clinical behavior and electroencephalographic epileptic activity has been studied in different animal models for focal and generalized epilepsy [1–4]. Results of these animal studies led to the development of an implantable device for human use and the first human trials for the treatment of epilepsy. The basis of vagus nerve stimulation for control of seizures is that vagal afferents have diffuse projections into the central nervous system and that activation of these afferents has a widespread effect on neuronal excitability [5]. The precise mechanism of action remains to be elucidated. Five acute-phase clinical studies (E01 to E05) involving the NCP System have been conducted in a total population of 454 patients (Table 1) [6–9]. Treatment with VNS reduces seizure frequency with at least 50% in 25–30% of patients. Long-term data were collected on all available E01 through E05 study patients [10]. Follow-up in these patients was between 1 and 3 years. Seventy-two percent of patients remained on the therapy. Over time an increase in the number of patients with a >50% reduction in seizure frequency was observed. There was a decrease of side effects such as hoarseness and voice change during stimulation over time. No clinically significant abnormalities of laboratory tests, ECG-Holter or pulmo-

Table 1. *Acute Clinical Studies with Vagus Nerve Stimulation*

Study	EO1	EO2	EO4	EO3	EO5
Type of study	Pilot longitudinal	Pilot longitudinal	Open longitudinal	Randomized parallel high/low	Randomized parallel High/low
Number of patients stimulated	10	5	123	115	198
Seizure type	partial	partial	all types	partial	partial
Number of AEDs	1–2	1–2	not specified	0–3	1–3
Mean reduction in seizures/day	24%	40%	7%	24% high/6% low	28% high/15% low
% of patients with >50% response	30%	50%	29%	30% high/14% low	23% high/16% low

AED Antiepileptic drug; *high* high stimulation mode; *low* low stimulation mode.

nary functioning testing occurred. A small percentage of patients became entirely seizure free [11].

The Neurocybernetic Prosthesis (NCP™) system is programmed to produce chronic, intermittent electrical pulses to the left vagus nerve requiring no intervention of the patient (programmed stimulation). This represents an advantage for uncooperative, noncompliant or mentally retarded patients. However, by moving a hand-held magnet over the device, additional electrical stimulation trains can be provided by the patient or caregiver in case of an aura or a seizure (magnet-induced stimulation) [12]. The purpose of this paper is to present the experience with VNS at Ghent University Hospital, Belgium and, in particular, to report the clinical efficacy of programmed and magnet induced stimulation.

Patients and Methods

Patients

Between March 1995 and June 2000, 30 patients (16 F, 14 M) with a mean age of 30 years (range: 12–69 years) and mean duration of refractory complex partial epilepsy of 18 years (range: 4–35 years) were treated with VNS. Mean follow-up in these patients was 33 months (range: 4–67 months). Patient characteristics are summarized in Table 2.

All patients underwent a comprehensive presurgical evaluation including video-EEG monitoring, optimum MRI, interictal FDG-PET and neuropsychological evaluation. They were considered unsuitable candidates for resective epilepsy surgery either because a single epileptogenic zone could not be defined or because of fear of postoperative deficits as suggested by the Wada-test or the location of underlying structural abnormalities in eloquent cortical areas. All patients were fully informed about the procedure and possible side effects and signed an informed consent.

Implantation Procedure

Stimulation of the vagus nerve is facilitated by implantation of the Neurocybernetic Prosthesis (NCP™) System (Cyberonics Inc., Houston Texas) which comprises a pulse generator and bipolar helical lead with an integral tether. The surgical procedure that has been described previously was performed under general anaesthesia during a 2-day admission at the neurosurgical department [13]. Intraoperatively generator circuitry and lead impedance was tested. The generator was activated 2 weeks postoperatively according to standard stimulation parameters (frequency: 30 Hz; pulse width: 500 µs; on time: 30 s; off time: 300 s). Output current was gradually increased with 0.25–0.5 mA increments every 2 weeks up to clinical efficacy or individual patient tolerance. At the time output current of the stimulator reached 1 mA all patients were provided with a magnet. Patients and caregivers were instructed on how to use the magnet in case of an aura or a seizure. Magnet output current was programmed 0.25 mA higher than the output current of the stimulator (frequency: 30 Hz, pulse width: 500 µs, on time: 60 s). The NCP™ software automatically logged the exact date and time when additional stimulation trains were delivered.

Table 2. *Patient Characteristics*

Patient n°	Patient initials	Sex	Age	Seizure duration (years)	Follow-up (months)	History	Seizure type
1	UP	M	33	22	67	febrile seizures, head trauma	CPS + SG
2	VD	F	30	4	67	head trauma	CPS ± SG/SPS
3	BI	M	35	12	61	head trauma	CPS ± SG
4	VC	F	29	18	59	encephalitis	CPS ± SG
5	SP	M	30	18	54	premature birth, callosotomy	CPS ± SG/SPS
6	HF	M	19	18	54	febrile seizures	CPS + SG
7	VE	M	27	22	53	head trauma	CPS ± SG
8	BI	F	21	18	47	febrile seizures, head trauma	CPS ± SG/SPS
9	JMA	F	31	9	44	febrile seizures	CPS ± SG
10	BJ	F	24	23	42	febrile seizures, encephalitis	CPS ± SG
11	GL	F	38	30	40	forceps birth	CPS ± SG
12	VJC	F	43	35	36	meningitis	CPS + SG
13	MG	F	16	11	36	none	CPS ± SG/SPS
14	VS	F	24	13	35	none	CPS ± SG
15	VC	M	20	6	31	meningitis, head trauma	CPS
16	MY	M	38	20	28	none	CPS ± SG
17	DK	M	12	5	26	none	CPS ± SG
18	HH	F	39	16	25	meningitis	CPS ± SG
19	BG	M	28	16	24	meningitis	CPS
20	DA	F	44	23	22	febrile seizures, meningitis	CPS ± SG
21	PH	M	36	30	22	encephalitis	CPS
22	VBP	M	49	35	21	febrile seizures	CPS
23	BM	F	41	19	19	none	CPS
24	PK	M	35	13	19	head trauma	CPS + SG
25	BL	F	26	25	18	LGS, corpus callosotomy	CPS ± SG
26	DK	F	28	25	14	none	CPS ± SG
27	CN	F	26	24	11	lennox-Gastaut syndrome	CPS ± SG
28	DVP	M	37	23	11	birth trauma	CPS
29	VA	F	22	16	8	left temporal astrocytoma	CPS
30	HT	M	24	6	4	cystic lesion left hemisphere	CPS + SG

CPS Complex partial seizures; *SG* secondary generalization; *SPS* simple partial seizures; *LGS* Lennox-Gastaut syndrome.

Data Collection

Patients were given a seizure diary and asked to provide a detailed account of their seizure frequency and severity and their use of the magnet. Patients were seen every month for further follow-up. Based on information reported by the patient seizure frequency, seizure type, prescribed AEDs and dosage as well as side effects of VNS were assessed at every clinic visit. Patients were also questioned about the dates and times when they used the magnet and about what they thought was the result of the additional stimulation train(s). Using the NCP™ software logged magnet use was verified and correlated with the patient's seizure diary.

Patients in whom discrepancies between logged and reported magnet use were found more than once per month were considered to be unreliable and excluded from the analysis. Patients in whom relatives and/or caregivers were not able to confirm reported seizure frequency were also excluded from further analysis.

A positive effect of magnet use was defined as a sudden interruption of seizures at the stage of the aura or later on during the habitual course regardless whether this occurred consistently at every instance or occasionally.

Mean monthly complex partial seizure frequency during the year before and the full follow-up period after the day of implantation were compared using the Wilcoxon signed-rank test (WSRT). For the purpose of this study responders were defined as patients who experienced a seizure frequency reduction of >50%; patients with a seizure frequency reduction of ≤50% were considered to be non-responders.

Results

Mean monthly complex partial seizure frequency changed from 34 (range: 2–200) to 11 (range: 0–60) (p = 0.0028; WSRT). Fourteen patients (47%) had a

Table 3. *Efficacy and Side Effects*

Patient n°	CPS frequency/ month before VNS	CPS frequency/ month after VNS	Output current (mA)	SG after VNS	Side effects
1	8	1	2.25	yes	unpleasant throat sensation
2	3	0	1.5	no	none
3	4	0	1.5	no	none
4	40	20	2.75	yes	none
5	4	3	2.5	yes	none
6	4	1	2.5	yes	none
7	30	20	2	yes	none
8	4	0	1.5	no	none
9	16	5	2.25	yes	hoarseness
10	35	20	2.75	yes	none
11	8	4	2.75	yes	hoarseness
12	2	0	1.75	no	none
13	200 (clusters)	0	1.25	no	none
14	30	20	1	yes	hoarseness
15	4	1	2.75	no	none
16	30	20	2.5	yes	none
17	12	9	2.25	no	shortness of breath
18	3	0	1.75	no	none
19	30	20	2.25	no	none
20	10	5	1.5	no	none
21	4	2	2.75	no	hoarseness
22	30	15	1.75	no	none
23	15	4	2	no	hoarseness
24	4	2	2	no	none
25	180	60	1.5	yes	none
26	150	60	1.75	yes	none
27	90	3	1.5	no	none
28	30	30	2.5	no	hoarseness
29	10	10	2.5	no	none
30	2	1	1.75	yes	none

CPS Complex partial seizures; *SG* secondary generalization; *VNS* vagus nerve stimulation; *mA* milliampères.

more than 50% reduction of seizure frequency. Six patients (20%) became free of complex partial seizures; two of them continue to experience simple partial seizures. Ten patients (33%) stopped having generalized tonic clonic seizures. Sixteen patients (53%) were non-responders. Mean follow-up was 33 months (range: 6–67). Mean maximal output current was 2 mA (range: 1 mA–2.75 mA). Table 3 shows the clinical efficacy data in the individual patients.

No peri-operative morbidity was reported. One patient had a surgical wound infection requiring antibiotic therapy during a one-week period. Shortness of breath, unpleasant sensation in the throat or hoarseness during the stimulation on-time were the most frequently reported chronic side effects, respectively in 1, 1 and 6 patients. None of the patients dropped out because of side effects; no devices had to be explanted.

In 2 patients gross discrepancies between reported and logged magnet use suggested that the reported information was unreliable. Three patients became seizure free before the magnet was provided. Six patients were unable to apply the magnet because there was no aura, seizures were too brief or caregivers unavailable. Eighteen out of thirty patients used the magnet and provided reliable information. In 6/18 patients (33%) no effect of the magnet was reported. Twelve out of 18 patients (66%) reported a positive effect of magnet use. Two of these patients were able to consistently abort CPS themselves. In 12/18 patients the magnet was commonly applied by a caregiver. This allowed to abort both CPS (n = 11) and generalized seizures (n = 2). Seven out of 12 patients who benefited from magnet use ultimately became responders. Table 4 shows individual patient data on the reported use and efficacy of magnet stimulation.

Table 4. *Use and Efficacy of Additional Magnet Stimulation*

Patient n°	Unreliable information	Use by patient	Use by caregiver	No response	Response	Effect on CPS	Effect on SG
1		−	−				
2		+		+			
3		−	−				
4		−	−				
5	+						
6		−	−				
7		+	−	+			
8		−	−				
9		+	−		+	+	
10		−	+		+	−	+
11	+						
12		−	−				
13		−	−				
14		−	−				
15		−	+		+	+	
16		+	−	+			
17		−	+		+	+	
18		−	+		+	+	+
19		−	+	+			
20		−	−				
21		−	+		+	+	
22		−	+		+	+	
23		−	+		+	+	
24	+		−		+	+	
25		−	+		+	+	
26		−	+		+	+	
27		−	+		+	+	
28	+		−	+			
29		−	+	+			
30		−	−				

CPS Complex partial seizures, *SG* secondary generalization.

Discussion

VNS is an effective alternative treatment for patients with refractory epilepsy who are unsuitable candidates for resective epilepsy surgery. Programmed with standard stimulation parameters the NCP™ device stimulates chronically and intermittently without patient intervention. Battery life reaches 5 years with intermittent stimulation; continuous stimulation is incompatible with reasonable battery life. Several studies have demonstrated the persistence of a stimulation effect after discontinuation of the stimulation train [14–16]. In this study we intended to evaluate the clinical efficacy of vagus nerve stimulation both in the programmed intermittent stimulation mode and magnet stimulation mode.

Patients, companions and caregivers were instructed on how to administer additional stimulation trains when an aura or a seizure onset occurred. We assumed that patients or caregivers could recognize habitual seizures and were able to evaluate sudden interruption of these seizures. In 63% of patients who were able to self-administer or receive additional magnet stimulation seizures could be interrupted, be it consistently or occasionally. This finding should be interpreted with some caution. Our data collection was mainly based on reporting by patients and caregivers. When data reported by the patients or caregivers in a seizure diary matched the information recorded by the NCP™ software we considered this to be reliable. Still, some patients may have under- or overreported seizure frequency. More specifically, patients who experienced isolated auras before VNS may have overestimated the seizure aborting effect of additional magnet stimulation trains when these auras occurred after the device was implanted.

More than half of the patients who reported a positive effect of magnet stimulation became responders.

For these patients the magnet feature of the device was a helpful tool to improve seizure control. Only two patients were able to use the magnet themselves. In most cases support from caregivers was necessary.

Different studies have shown that vagus nerve stimulation is an efficacious but palliative treatment for patients with refractory epilepsy [6–9]. Our efficacy results, showing a responder rate of 47% from programmed stimulation, compare favorably with the current consensus in the literature. It is generally accepted that at least 1/3 of patients have an improvement in seizure control with a reduction in seizure frequency of at least 50%, 1/3 of patients experience a worthwhile reduction of seizure frequency between 30 and 50%. In the remaining 1/3 of the patients there is little or no effect.

To our knowledge, this study is the first to explore the efficacy of magnet-induced vagus nerve stimulation. Our results suggest that the magnet is a useful tool that provides patients and mainly caregivers with an additional means of controlling refractory seizures. Additional controlled studies comparing programmed stimulation and magnet induced stimulation in monitoring conditions are warranted.

Acknowledgments

Part of the work presented in this article is supported by grant BOZF 01105399 from Ghent University. Dr. VONCK is sponsored by a junior researcher ("Aspirant") grant from the Fund for Scientific Research – Flanders. Prof. Dr. BOON is sponsored by grant 1.5.236.99 from the Fund for Scientific Research – Flanders.

References

1. Zanchetti A, Wang SC, Moruzzi G (1952) The effect of vagal afferent stimulation on the EEG pattern of the cat. Electroencephalog Clin Neurophysiol 4: 357–361

2. Zabara J (1992) Inhibition of experimental seizures in canines by repetitive stimulation. Epilepsia 33(6): 1005–1012

3. Woodbury DM, Woodbury JW (1990) Effects of vagal stimulation on experimentally induced seizures in rats. Epilepsia 31 [Suppl] 2: 7–19

4. Lockard JS, Congdon WC, DuCharme LL (1990) Feasibility and safety of vagal stimulation in monkey model. Epilepsia 31 [Suppl] 2: 20–26

5. Rutecki P (1990) Anatomical, pyhsiological and theoretical basis for the antiepileptic effect of vagus nerve stimulation. Epilepsia 31 [Suppl] 2: S1–S6

6. Handforth A, DeGorgio CM, Schachter SC et al (1998) Vagus nerve stimulation therapy for partial onset seizures. A randomized, active control trial. Neurology 51: 48–55

7. Ben-Menachem E, Manon-Espaillat R, Ristanovic R et al (1994) Vagus nerve stimulation for treatment of partial seizures: 1. A controlled study of effect on seizures. Epilepsia 35: 616–626

8. Ramsay RE, Uthman BM, Augustinsson LE et al (1994) Vagus nerve stimulation for treatment of partial seizures: 2. Safety, side-effects and tolerability. Epilepsia 35: 627–636

9. George R, Sonnen A, Upton A et al (1995) The Vagus Nerve Stimulation Study Group. A randomized controlled trial of chronic vagus nerve stimulation for treatment of medically intractable seizures. Neurology 45: 224–230

10. Morris GL, Mueller WM and the vagus nerve stimulation study group EO1–EO5 (1999) Long-term treatment with vagus nerve stimulation in patients with refractory epilepsy. Neurology 53(8): 1731–1735

11. Vonck K, Boon P, D'Havé M, Vandekerckhove T, O'Connor S, De Reuck J (1999) Long-term results of vagus nerve stimulation in refractory epilepsy. Seizure 8: 328–334

12. Reese T, Brent T, Zabara J (1990) An implantable neurocybernetic prosthesis system. Epilepsia 31 [Suppl] 2: S33–S37

13. Landy HJ, Ramsay RE, Slater J, Casiano RR, Morgan R (1993) Vagus nerve stimulation for complex partial seizures: surgical technique, safety and efficacy. J Neurosurg 78: 26–31

14. Lockard JS, Congdon WC, DuCharme LL (1990) Feasability and safety of vagal stimulation: the monkey model. Epilepsia 3 [Suppl] 2: S20–26

15. Takaya M, Terry WJ, Naritoku DK (1996) Vagus nerve stimulation induces a sustained anticonvulsant effect. Epilepsia 37: 1111–1116

16. McLaghlan RS (1993) Suppression of interictal spikes and seizures by stimulation of the vagus nerve. Epilepsia 34(5): 918–923

Correspondence: Prof. Dr. Paul Boon, M.D., Ph.D., Reference Center for Refractory Epilepsy, Ghent University Hospital, 185 De Pintelaan; B-9000 Gent, Belgium.

Acta Neurochir (2001) [Suppl] 79: 99–104

Computer Added Locomotion by Implanted Electrical Stimulation in Paraplegic Patients (SUAW)

K. von Wild[1], **P. Rabischong**[2], **G. Brunelli**[3], **M. Benichou**[4], and **K. Krishnan**[5]

[1] Neurosurgical Department and Unit for Early Neurorehabilitation, Clemenshospital, Teaching Hospital of the Medical University Münster, Germany
[2] Faculty of Medicine of Montpellier, Centre Propara Montpellier, France Fondazione Montecatone Rehabilitation Institute, Imola, Italy
[3] Fondazione Recerca Midolle Spinale, Brescia, Italy
[4] Centre Propara, Montpellier, France
[5] European Calies Association, University of Salford, UK

Summary

Paraplegia means a live long sentence of sensory loss, paralysis and dependence with approximately 1000 new victims in every European country every year and 11.500 new traumatic SCI cases in the US. respectively. Sixty percent are injured before age 30. More than 90% of SCI victims may survive with nearly normal experience of live. Most patients will recover somewhat from SCI over time but no patient who remained plegic for one year regains voluntary motor function after that time period.

Despite remarkable efforts and recent achievements in rehabilitation no treatment can be recommended so far to enhance functional recovery and restoring locomotion in paraplegic humans. FES as a technical compensation has become therefore a challenging treatment to restore muscle function and to prevent atrophy and to improve mobility and quality of life at the same time. In paraplegics FES could be the basis to restore locomotion. One of the advantages of an implanted FES version (neuroprosthesis) is that the FES system, electrodes, and cables remain permanently implanted within the body, so that the patient can stay without cables, the programmer attached to the crutches.

The SUAW project, supported under BIOMED II Programme by the European Community was aimed to finalise and to put into practice the results of previous research and development. The novel implant with an ASCI-Chip has 16 channels, 8 on each side, 20 mA for monopolar and 2 mA for bipolar stimulation, only one electrode can be stimulated at a given time. Stimulation of 6 muscle groups of both legs are known to be sufficient for locomotion: M. ileopsoas (erector of the body, hip flexor), M. gluteus maximus (hip extensor), M. gluteus medius (lateral hip stabilisator, knee abductor), Mm. hamstrings (knee flexor) stimulated by epimysial electrodes, Mm. sartorius and rectus femoris (knee extensor) stimulated by neural, bipolar electrodes. Patient's selection criteria were: stable spinal cord lesion between T7 and T11, minimum 1 year after the accident without deformity of the spine, the muscle groups for locomotion responding to external FES with the EXOSTIM programmer with the same programme used later for the neuroprosthesis. Two paraplegic male patients, T8, 38 and 31 years old respectively, were operated on by an international group of surgeons according to the protocol in 09/1999, respectively 7/2000. The postop. course was uneventful. Because the threshold of the primary implant was too low regarding scare tissue around the electrodes, this implant was changed in 01/2000 and worked perfectly. Both patients are happy with the success of the novel treatment modalities.

Keywords: Spinal cord injury; paraplegia; neuroprosthesis; BIOMED II-Project.

Introduction

There are in Europe about 300.000 paraplegics and in every country approximately 1000 new cases per year with an increasing number of tetraplegics, due to the quality of both emergency care and early neurorehabilitation of the victims [1, 5–8]. We can differentiate a tetraplegia, impairing more or less all four limbs, and a paraplegia, immobilizing the lower limbs. A vertebral lesion, for example in T8 (eight thoracic vertebrae) produces a medullary deficiency corresponding to a medullar metameric segment located below while the voluntary function of the muscles above are preserved [2].

Sir Ludwig Guttman [7] and his vision on and practical experiences in acute treatment and early neurorehabilitation in paraplegic patients, trained by O. Foerster [6], changed completely the attitude of medical management in spinal cord injury (SCI). Achievements include better first aid, organized units for acute care and rehabilitation, precise diagnostic imaging (spiral CT, MRI), surgical techniques for decompression and fusion [8], better understanding of the pathophysiology [2, 6, 7] and management of complications [1, 5]. Although many promising treatments in laboratory animals are reported, including surgical reconstructive procedures, non has so far been proven a standard procedure to enhance neurological recovery in humans [1, 4, 5, 12, 13]. Regarding neurorehabilitation functional electrical stimulation (FES) became an important pillar [10, 11].

The implanted FES version which we call neuroprosthesis [14] has the advantages that the electronic stimulation system and the electrodes are permanently implanted within the body, so that no gluing of electrodes onto the skin and cables will hinder the patient during the exercises while he is carrying the antenna which sends the power and the signal of the portable programmer, preparing the right stimulation sequences. In America NeuroControl, Cleveland, USA has already performed more than 100 implantations of free hand neuroprosthesis, including in Europe on tetraplegic patients [9, 10] and first results with implanted FES for mobility in paraplegic are promising [5, 11].

The purpose of this project was to demonstrate in paraplegics adequate normal like walking performance and the possibility to stand up by voluntary artificial FES of 6 muscle groups in both legs with the aid of only one novel designed neuroprosthesis.

Material and Methods

On August 1st 1996 the European community project "SUAW" (Table 1) was started, co-ordinated by P. R., which ended in June 2000, (Tab. 1). The project was evaluated by the Ethical Committees of the Universities of Montpellier and Bologna with permission for implantation of the novel neuroprosthesis in human paraplegics.

The work of the project was subdivided into 6 tasks as follows

1) Selection of patients including medical examination, physical and biomechanical assessments, Magnetic Resonance Imaging (MRI) and/or CT Scanning.

Including criteria were a stable spinal lesion T7–T11, minimum of one year after the lesion with a reasonable acceptance of the situation and good understanding of the residual complications of paraplegia. The subjects had to be functionally independent. Lack of spine de-

Table 1. *SUAW – Partners*

1. Neuromedics, Montpellier, France, Mr. Bernard Denis, co-ordinator of the industrial partners IBM France, Thomson CSF, Neuromedics in France, and Roessingh R & D in The Netherlands.
2. University of Salford, Manchester, UK: Prof. Jack Edwards and Prof. Kris Krishnan co-ordinator of the scientific, medical, and surgical work.
3. Six clinic centres: Copenhagen/Alborg, Denmark, Montpellier, France, Münster/Bad Wildungen, Germany, Bologna/Montecantone, Italy, Enschede, The Netherlands, Southport, United Kingdom.

Table 2. *Muscles to React Positively During Stimulation for Gait Functions*

Hip extensor – m. gluteus maximus.
Hip flexors – m. satorius, m. rectus femoris
lateral hip stabilisator – Knee abductor and m. gluteus medius.
Knee extensor – m. quadriceps
Knee flexor – m. hamstrings (m. biceps femoral, m. semitendinouse, and semimembranouse)
Foot extensor – m. tibialis antèrior
During stimulation the patient should not feel any pain and unpleasant sensations.

formity. Patients' age between 18 and 60, patients' weight should not be more than 15% above normal body weight calculated by kg per cm high above 100 cm. Muscle groups (Tab. 2) must respond to cutaneous electrical stimulation, having been tested and trained with the aid of an EXOSTIM stimulator (Neuromedics) with the same programme used later for the neuroprosthesis.

Most important: the patient must be motivated to go into this difficult and complex process in all to restore an upright position and locomotion during the next years.

Contraindications were contracture and hypermobility specially of the knee and hip and spasticity interfering with the stimulation of predetermined muscles and the lower limbs. Body overweight.

2) Pre-surgical training of selected patients, duration 12 weeks.

As a result of prolonged post-injury desuse, muscle of paraplegic patients tend to lose their capacity for generating contraction force. The effects of this so-called atrophy must be reversed by specific (FES) muscle training.

At least two French and two Italien patients were selected for the first implantation in 1999.

3) Prototype Manufacturing of the FES Package with an implantable part of the electronic box (Fig. 1), electrodes (Fig. 2a–b, 3a–b), cables, connectors and with the portable part of the antenna, programmer, command interface plus the surface stimulation for pre-surgical training phase Exostim (Neuromedics) and implant epimysial electrodes (Fraunhofer Institute) perineural electrodes (ARTROTECH).

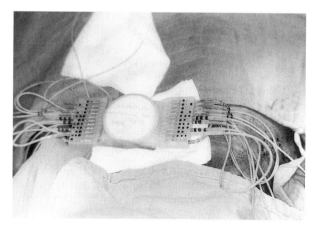

Fig. 1. Neuromedics® implant (70 mm⌀) contains the ASIC chip of 3.9 × 45 mm size with 70 wire pads bounded to a 9 × 9 mm ceramic packages. 8 output channels on both sides monopolar 20 mA (1.5 kΩ, bipolar 2 mA) threshold, here connected to the electrodes at the end of implantation of neuroprothesis

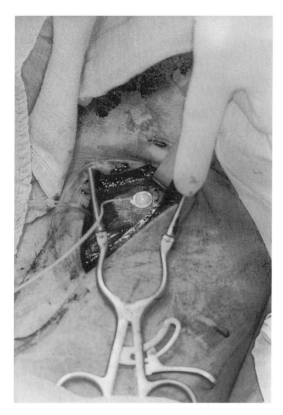

Fig. 2. Epimysial elecetrodes (Fraunhofer Institute®) to be fixed over the motor point of the gluteus muscle

4) Surgical Implantation, duration 2 weeks. The surgical protocol was accepted after a period of intensive discussion and training of the team.

The implants were tolerated without complications in animal experiences including primates at CICE of Clermont-Ferrand and the Anatomy Labs. of the Med. Faculties of Montpellier and Clermont Ferrand) including endoscopical techniques with novel Stortz® endoscope. All surgeons were experts in plastic reconstructive* and neurosurgery**. Michel Benichou, MD, Montpellier*, Prof. Giorgio Brunelli, MD, Bologna*, Prof. Krish Krishnan, MD, Salford**, Ole Osgaard, MD, Copenhagen*, Hans Van der AA, MD, Enschede**, Prof. Klaus R. H. von Wild, MD, Münster**, Bakul Soni, MD Southport**.

5) Post-surgical training, performed by the same experts in physiotherapy as preop, was scheduled for a duration of 12 weeks, after bed rest for 2 weeks.

Technical Remarks

The implant (Fig. 1) contains two types stimulation outputs: Monopolar for epimysial electrodes (Fig. 2) and bipolar for neural electrodes stimulation (Fig. 3), 16 output channels: monopolar 20 mA (1.5 KΩ) 2 mA bipolar, 8 channels available, on each side. Only one electrode can be stimulated at a given time.

The Neuromedics implant of 70 mm in diameter was specially designed for this project, contains the

novel ASIC chip (IBM-France Corbeil) with the size of 3.9 × 4.5 mm with 70 wire pads bounded to a 9 × 9 mm ceramic package.

Surgical Procedures

The first patient, Marc M., 38 years, paraplegic T8 after car accident in 1989 was operated on September 28th 1999 at Propara Hospital by M. B., G. B., K. v. W., assisted by the technical team and physiotherapists who were in charge of the Exostim FES programme and neuroprosthesis for verifying the muscular stimulation during surgery.

The procedure started with the patient wrapped in prone position (Fig. 4) with simultaneous approach on both dorsal sides and the setting of epimysial electrodes (Fig. 2) on the muscles surface at the motor point level on the mm. gluteus maximus and medius followed by the hamstrings and the neural electrode (Fig. 3) around the group of peroneus muscle fascicles of the sciatic nerve corresponding to the foot extensor muscle. After closure of the wounds the patient was turned around. In upright position the epimysial elec-

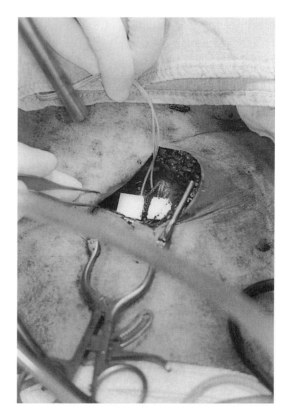

Fig. 3. Bipolar neural electrode (ARCROTECH®) around the muscle fibres of the peroneal nerve

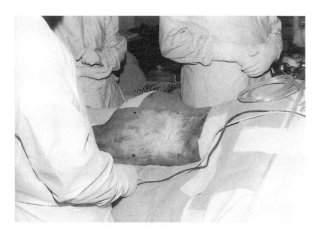

Fig. 4. Muscle points were marked on the skin according to pre-op. Exostim® stimulation were for the gluteus maximus, medius and the hamstrings with the patient in prone position

tient completed his postoperative rehabilitation followed by continuous physiotherapy. After one year of training with the aid of the new prosthesis he is now able to stand up and to walk on the ground up to 100 m supported by his arms and walking frame that will be changed to arm crutches.

The second patient, Ludovico S., 32 years old, paraplegic since a motor scooter accident 10 years before, was operated in the hospital of Imola, Italy by G. B., K. v. W., and M. B. on July 26th, 2000. The procedure was the same as the first one but the neuroprosthesis had the same characteristics like the second one we implanted. The 8 hour operation and postoperative course with following training in Montecantone were uneventful with so far promising results.

trodes were placed simultaneously on both sides on the iliopsoas muscle, one neural electrode on the muscular part of the femoral nerve by minimal invasive microsurgical and endoscopic techniques with aid of a Stortz® endoscope. The receiver was implanted into a supraumbilic subcutaneous pouch (Fig. 4). The total time of procedure was 12 hours because of long lasting process of electric stimulation of each electrode and physiological testing of each muscle before connecting.

At the end, however, when stimulating the epimysial electrodes at 10 mA, some perturbations appeared during the activation of the implant by the antenna inducing a stimulation of all four neural electrodes. After some weeks and encapsulation of the electrodes by normal scar tissue fibrosis the current intensity for stimulating the electrodes both epimysial (10 mA) and neural (0.2 mA) turned out to be too low according to the threshold of the receiver.

Therefore a second operation was performed for revision and exchange of the implant by M. B. and K. v. W. on February 14th, 2000.

All the neural electrodes in the range of 7 to 3 milliamp were answering positively. All the epimysial electrodes, except the one for the left medial gluteus muscle where positively activated at the range 7 to 25 milliamp. The impedance was in the order of 500 ohms for the epimysial's and of 2500 ohms for the neural's. Therefore the new implant with higher mA limits was connected and tested positively and the interference between neural and epimysial didn't exist any more. The postoperative course was uneventful and the pa-

Discussion

The only way of course to restore voluntary muscle command, sphincter functions for bladder and rectum evacuation control and cutaneous sensibility to localising in space the paralysed limbs is to bridge the gap of the spinal cord lesion by artificial regeneration at the nervous fibres level [2, 4, 8]. Because in the central nervous system the natural regeneration of nervous fibres after the transaction lesion is stopped after a couple of weeks by fibrosis process, mainly due to the oligodendrocytes, responsible for the manufacturing of myelinic tubes [13]. This process may be interpreted as a spinal cord auto-protection system to avoid chaotic and hazardous reconnections.

Although single case reports in human paraplegics may show promising results [1, 3, 4, 12, 13] FES by both external and implanted electrodes are still experimental [9–11]. Functional rehabilitation using all the modern facilities and techniques has demonstrated the real possibility to have a better control of the lesion, to activate compensatory mechanisms and to develop efficient rehabilitative procedures and so to achieve today an acceptable final outcome.

In fact those muscles under the spinal cord lesion are still alive even so they are not under brain control, they keep their contraction capacity, yet diminished, but clinically useably. Therefore (FES) has been used for a long time and is intensively used nowadays by many teams around the world to support and to restore artificial locomotion programmes in the lower limbs [5, 9–11]. The electrical current can be applied to the muscles in 6 different ways:

Table 3. *Clinical Application of FES*

1) Through the skin (cutaneous ES)
2) Directly in the muscle (intramuscular ES)
3) On the muscle surface (epimysial ES)
4) By electrodes placed around or inside the muscular nerve (neural ES)
5) Inside the spinal canal at the motor root levels (radicular ES)
6) Placed directly on the spinal cord (medullar ES)

There is neither an effective pharmacotherapy [1, 5] nor a combined therapy with biotechnology [12, 13] or a plastic reconstructive surgical technique available today [3, 4, 8] for human paraplegics to make them walking after a complete interruption of the spinal cord. Regeneration of lost neurons or axons in human SCI remains an unrealized goal [5].

The transfer of promising experimental data from animals, e.g. rats, to men is particularly difficult. The great differences lie in the neuronal organisation of the spinal cord [2], in which an interneuronal machinery is responsible for generating semi-automatic sequences of activation of the different spinal cord metamaric levels devoted to locomotion. In man this semiautomatic interneuronal machinery is more under the control of the brain, explaining the great diversity of movements and positions that man can archive consciously and voluntary [5–7]. These interneuronal mechanisms are used today intensively in physical training of paraplegic patients, e.g. with the mechanised weight supported locomotion (treadmill, gait trainer) [5] while the body weight is supported with a modified parachute carrying belt and the central stimulating concept of non-use – forced use, which was already postulated by O. Foerster 1916 [6].

Implanted FES for computer added locomotion in paraplegia was demonstrated to be possible and effective in humans according to the limited results of implanted patients reported in the literature. Restoring locomotion for walking in paraplegia by means of FES has been investigated intensively for the last 30 years [9–11]. The idea is to co-ordinate the actions of the paralysed muscle groups by delivering sequences of electrical pulses trough a network of electrodes either attached to the surface of the body or implanted target to allow the paraplegic patient to stand up and to walk by artificial stimulation. Regarding upright mobility and walking functional anatomy shows that 6 muscles stimulated according to physiological movement may be enough [10]: a.) Two channels bilaterally for bipolar

neural stimulation of the femoral nerve muscle fibres of the quadriceps to cause knee extension and two for the muscular part of the ischiatic nerve to induce withdrawal reflex causing simultaneous activation of hip and knee flexures; b.) Epimysial monopolar electrodes placed dorsal over the motor points for activation of gluteus maximus (hip extensor), gluteus medius (lateral hip stabilisator and knee abductor), and to the hamstrings (knee flexors: the biceps femoral, semitendinous and semimembranous), ventral to the hip flexor m. ileopsoas, which is the important muscle for erection of the body. Implantable systems available for clinical application were so far generally limited to 8 channels because of the stimulators' size and therefore normally two implants per person were used [11]. An eight channel stimulator for percutaneous stimulation is meanwhile widely used in physiotherapy to prevent atrophy of the muscles in paraplegics and at the same time to relieve the body weight while the arms are carrying the body weight during transfer. Muscles artificially stimulated with up to 48 channels are reported to result in improved speed and stability of gate and the ability to do side stepping and stair climbing [9]. According to Kobetic *et al.* stimulation of the peroneal nerve for dorsi-flexion may be accompanied by some flexion reflex which had a balancing effect or enhanced the response of direct stimulation of the hip flexors. We designed a 14 channel combined stimulation with 4 neural and 10 epimysial electrodes in respect to functional anatomy regarding "Stand up and Walk" procedure with only one novel implant of 70 mm size. Our results obtained during the follow up were comparable with the results reported during the 8 channel Exostim with surface stimulation and are in agreement with those published in the literature.

Our neuroprosthesis was very well tolerated according to our animal experimental studies before implantation in humans. Normal fibrosis reaction of the tissues around the electrodes turned out to create a biological encapsulation with slight increase of the threshold seen in acute preparations, so that with 2 milliAm for neural and 20 milliAm for epimysial electrodes no electronic "noise" in the radio frequency transmission has been observed anymore in both of our patients during the follow up. Following the surgical protocol using minimal invasive microsurgical dissection and endoscopy no complication has been observed during our operative procedures in both patients including the revision with exchange of the receiver in the first patient.

The designed concept became a challenging task for neurosurgeons when working together in a transdisciplinary neurorehabilitation team targeted to restoration of locomotion. Our project was awarded with an *Inscription into the Golden Book of the European Community* because of the success of the SUAW project.

References

1. Braken MB, Shepard MJ, Holford TR *et al* (1997) Administration of methylprednisolone for 24 or 48 hours or tirilazad mesylate for 48 hours in the treatment of acute spinal cord injury. JAMA, May 28 277(20): 1597–1604
2. Brown AG (1981) Oganization in the spinal cord. The anatomy and physiology of identified neurones. Springer, Berlin Heidelberg New York
3. Brunelli GA, Brunelli GR (1999) Restoration of walking in paraplegia by transferring the ulnar nerve to the hip: a report on the first patient. Microsurgery 19: 223–226
4. Carlstedt T, Grane P, Hallin RG *et al* (1999) Return of function after spinal cord implantation of avulsed spinal nerve roots. Lancet 346: 1323–1325
5. Dietz V (1996) Querschnittslähmung. Kohlhammer, Stuttgart
6. Foerster O (1916) Therapie der Motilitätsstörungen bei Erkrankungen des Zentralnervensystems. In: Vogt H (Hrsg) Handbuch der Therapie der Nervenkrankheiten, Bd. 2. Symptomatische Therapie der Organneurosen. Krankheitsbilder und deren Behandlung. Fischer, Jena, S860–940
7. Guttmann L (1960) Rehabilitation (with special references to spinal paraplegia) Rev Int Serv Santé Armées 33: 60
8. Kim YS, Cho YE, Chin DK *et al* (2000) Advances in the surgical management of spinal cord injury. RNNEEL 16(3,4): 190–191
9. Kobetic R, Carroll SG, Marsolaise EB (1986) Paraplegic stair climbing assisted by electrical stimulation. Proc. 39Th ACEMB Conf, Baltimore, MD, p 256
10. Kobetic R, Triolo RJ, Marsolais EB (1997) Muscle selection and walking performance of multichannel FES systems for ambulation in paraplegia. IEEE Transactions on Rehabilitation Engineering 5: 23–29
11. Kobetic R, Tirolo RJ, Uhlir JP *et al* (1999) Implanted functional electric stimulation system for mobility in paraplegia: A follow-up case report. IEEE Transactions on Rehabilitation Engineering 7(4): 390–398
12. Kojima A, Tator CH (2000) Intrathecal administration of epidermal growth factor and fibroblast growth factor 2 promotes ependymal proliferation and functional recovery after spinal cord injury in adult rats. RNNEEL 16(3,4): 150–151
13. Schwab M (2000) Regeneration, reorganization and repair in spinal cord injury. RNNEEL 16(3,4): 189–190
14. Pedotti AM, Ferrarin J, Quintern R Riener (eds) (1996) Neuroprosthesis from basic research to clinical applications. Springer, Berlin Heidelberg New York Tokyo

Correspondence: Prof. Dr. med. Klaus von Wild, Clinic of Neurosurgery with Department of Neurorehabilitation, Clemenshospital, Düesbergweg 124, D-48153 Münster, Germany.

Acta Neurochir (2001) [Suppl] 79: 105–107

Application of a Dual Channel Peroneal Nerve Stimulator in a Patient with a "Central" Drop Foot

H. E. van der Aa[1,2]**, G. Bultstra**[3]**, A. J. Verloop**[3]**, L. Kenney**[4]**, J. Holsheimer**[3]**, A. Nene**[4]**, H. J. Hermens**[4]**, G. Zilvold**[3,4]**, and H. P. J. Buschman**[2]

[1] Department of Neurosurgery, Enschede, The Netherlands
[2] Twente Institute for Neuromodulation (TWIN), Medisch Spectrum Twente, The Netherlands
[3] Roessingh Research & Development, Enschede, The Netherlands
[4] Technical University, Enschede, The Netherlands

Summary

Dropped foot is a common mobility problem amongst patients after a cerebro vascular accident. The condition arises from paresis of the muscles that control the foot movement during the swing phase of gait. If the abnormal movement is not compensated for, it results in a significant decrease in the mobility and hence quality of life.

Compensation for the drop foot can be achieved through the application of functional electrical stimulation. To date, in the clinical environment, the stimulation has been applied through electrodes placed on the skin over the common peroneal nerve, and using a single channel implant device. It is well known that with these techniques it is difficult to establish a balanced response of the foot.

An implantable dual channel system for stimulation of the deep and superficial peroneal nerve has now been developed for patients with a drop foot following a stroke. By stimulation of the two branches of the common peroneal nerve separately it is possible to achieve a precisely balanced dorsal flexion and eversion of the foot. Stimulation occurs via small bipolar electrodes which are placed subepineural. After successful tests on animals we have now started the two channel peroneal nerve stimulator implantation in patients. The preliminary results of the first implants are presented.

Keywords: Implant; drop foot; function restoration; functional electrical stimulation.

Introduction

Functional electrical stimulation (FES) systems for the treatment of dropped foot are now in clinical use in significant numbers. Compared with the use of orthosis electrical stimulation has a number of advantages: it prevents muscle atrophy, the blood flow remains normal or even improves and it is cosmetically better accepted. FES can be applied especially in patients with an unimpaired peripheral nerve system. This is because it is much more convenient, with respect to functionality and energy efficiency to stimulate nerves, rather than stimulate muscles directly. The interface between the nerves and the stimulator consists of the electrode. Two different approaches for FES are being studied. The oldest technique is surface stimulation, which means that electrodes that are placed on the skin electrically activate the muscles by depolarising the innervating nerves that run subcutaneous. The second technique uses implanted electrodes.

Surface stimulation is applied in most cases. However, both the quality of treatment and scope of application are limited by factors inherent to any surface system [2]. Examples of these are repeated difficulty in locating the correct points for stimulation, difficulty in reaching the deeper lying nerves, lack of selectivity, variation in skin impedance and electrode position makes resetting of pulse-amplitude necessary, physical discomfort experienced by the patient, and low efficiency of the energy used for activation of the nerve. Recognition of these limitations has led to several attempts to produce a clinically useful implantable system.

Initially single channel implant devices were tested [3], [4]. A major technical problem encountered was the lack of selectivity associated with the electrode siting. The electrodes were attached to the common peroneal nerve, the same nerve that is stimulated by the surface devices. The placement of the electrodes during surgery to produce the desired movement of the foot was achievable. However, the response during walking was usually very different from that under surgery due to the loading of the ankle, day-to-day changes in calf tone and inevitable small changes in the electrode-nerve interface properties. These changes could not be compensated for with a single channel system and therefore, this approach failed [5]. One solution to this lack of flexibility is to increase the number of electrode sites to two, attached to the two branches of the peroneal nerve. It is proposed that this approach will hold two advantages over existing methods. Firstly, it will provide greater selectivity over the resulting motion. Secondly, by allowing the ratio of stimulation to the two branches to be adjusted, it should provide the flexibility to compensate for changes in the neuromuscular system that may occur over time.

A system based on this approach was designed and developed by our group [1]. The first peroneal nerve stimulators were recently implanted in two patients. Here we present preliminary results obtained with this system.

Methods and Results

The stimulator system consists of four parts: the receiver-stimulator, the transmitter, the foot switch and the charger. The implantable 2-channel peroneal nerve stimulator is shown in Figure 1. The receiver is a passive device, receiving information carried by the radio frequency signals and converting them to the stimulation pulses of the desired amplitude and frequency. It is secured under the skin on the lateral side of the affected leg by sutures through locating tabs. The stimulation pulses are passed from the receiver along a pair of leads to the two electrode sets, one located under the epineurium of the superficial peroneal nerve, the other located under the epineurium of the deep peroneal nerve. The implanted receiver is being produced by the University Twente and Finetech-Medical (Welwyn

Garden City, Hertsfortshire, England), a company with many years experience with the production of the Finetech-Brindley bladder stimulator.

The stimulation ratio of the two channels is set by the user or clinician at the start of use. The stimulation is triggered by recognition of "heel off", as detected by a switch located under the heel of the patient (Figure 2A and B). After a fixed delay, the stimulation pulse current is ramped up on both channels to the two levels corresponding to the setting on the two knobs on the transmitter. Stimulation continues at 30 Hz, with a pulse duration of 0.3 msec during the swing phase. Following detection of heel strike, stimulation continues for a fixed time and is then ramped down to zero on both channels.

The transmitter is shown in Figure 2B. The function of the transmitter is to generate the required stimulation signals at appropriate points in time and to transmit these signals on radio frequency carrier waves to the implanted receiver. The design approach taken in the new stimulator uses a single transmission coil whose transmission frequency oscillates between the natural frequencies of the two receiver coils. This has the effect of multiplexing the signals. As only a single transmission coil is required, this can be made relatively large when compared with the diameters of the receiving coils and hence the link is relatively tolerant of misalignment. The transmitter is housed in a box of height 100 mm, width 50 mm, and depth 20 mm, weighing approximately 0.1 kg. The transmitter is attached with straps on the lateral side of the lower leg, over the site of the implant, just below the knee. The footswitch provides information to the transmitter for timing purposes.

The charger (not shown) is a simple transformer, converting the mains supply to the voltage required to recharge the batteries in the transmitter. A charged battery has sufficient power to be used all day. Recharging of the batteries is done overnight.

Results and Discussion

Two patients, both with a drop foot as a result of a cerebral vascular accident and a stable neurology for at least one year, were implanted with the device. In both patients during the implantation, good functional dorsiflexion and eversion movements were obtained

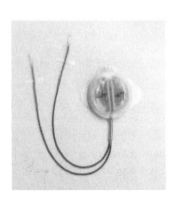

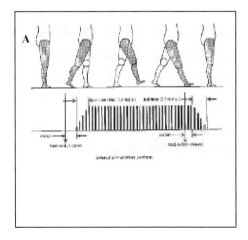

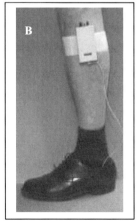

Fig. 1. Implantable 2-channel receiver-stimulator. ∅: 33 mm

Fig. 2. (A) Stimulation pattern. (B) Transmittor mounted on lower leg above the implanted receiver-stimulator. A heel-switch activates the stimulation timing

with electrical stimulation of the deep and superficial peroneal branches, respectively. Ten days after implantation the wound was checked, neurophysiological measurements were performed to test nerve integrity, and therapy was started. The first implanted patient, who experienced physical discomfort and skin problems with surface stimulation is now free of any surface stimulation induced pain and skin problems. The measurements that were performed consisted of optimisation of the stimulation settings in each of the two channels individually, and of the two channels when used simultaneously. This was performed during isometric torque measurements of the foot, and during gait analysis in the gait lab. From the first implanted subject we have data from four repeated measurements with one week interval. From the second subject at present we do not have sufficient follow-up data to be included here. The distance that the first subject could walk in 6 minutes was increased by about 40% the first time after implantation when compared to preimplantation, and slightly increased further with repeated measurements. These measurements also showed that the stimulation output (voltage) remained stable, indicating that the electrode-nerve interface did not change over time. This means that the nerve integrity is preserved, the position of the electrode with respect to the nerve did not vary, and there was no connective tissue growth between electrode and nerve. There was a linear relation between stimulation output and the functional movement (as measured in force) both for dorsiflexion and eversion, indicating that stimulation output and functional movement can be adjusted easily by the subjects themselves.

These preliminary results indicate that the use of a two channel peroneal nerve stimulator for restoration of a drop foot is safe and effective. Additional gait training and physiotherapy of these patients will further help improve their gait in time, which may eventually help to fully restore their functionality.

References

1. Holsheimer J et al (1993) Implantable dual channel peroneal nerve stimulator. Proc Ljubljana FES Conf: 42–44
2. Rushton DN (1997) Functional electrical stimulation. Physiol Meas 18: 241–275
3. Stronijk P et al (1987) Treatment of drop foot using an implantable peroneal underknee stimulator. Scand J Rehab 19: 37–43
4. Waters RL et al (1975) Experimental correction of footdrop by electrical stimulation of the peroneal nerve. J Bone Joint Surg 57A(8): 1047–1054
5. Waters RL et al (1985) Functional electrical stimulation of the peroneal nerve for hemiplegia. Long term clinical follow-up. J Bone Joint Surg 67-A: 792–793

Correspondence: H. E. van der Aa, Department of Neurosurgery, Medisch Spectrum Twente, 7500 KA, The Netherlands.

Acta Neurochir (2001) [Suppl] 79: 109–111

Rehabilitation of Hearing and Communication Functions in Patients with NF2

J. Kuchta, R. Behr, M. Walger, O. Michel, and **N. Klug**

Department of Neurosurgery and Department of ENT-Surgery, University of Cologne, Cologne, Germany

Summary

Most patients with neurofibromatosis type 2 (NF2) lose hearing either spontaneously or after removal of their neurofibromas. The patient may benefit from conventional hearing aids if, due to modern microsurgery and intraoperative monitoring the integrity of the cochlea and the 8th nerve is preserved. With lost auditory function but preserved electrical stimulability of the 8th nerve a cochlear implant may be appropriate. But if the patients have no remaining 8th nerve to stimulate, there is no benefit from cochlear implants. Until some years ago, vibrotactile aids, lip-reading, and sign language have been the only communication modes available to these patients.

With auditory brain stem implants it is now possible to bypass both the cochlea and the 8th nerve and to stimulate the cochlear nucleus directly. Stimulation of the devices produces useful auditory sensations in almost all patients. Testing of perceptual performance indicated significant benefit from the device for communication purposes, including sound-only sentence recognition scores and the ability to converse on the telephone. Also lip-reading is significantly improved with brain stem implants. The successful work of an auditory brainstem program center depends very much on the close interdisciplinary collaboration between the Departments of Neurosurgery and ENT-surgery. In the future new developments like speech processing strategies and new designed electrodes accessing the complex tonotopic organization of the cochlear nucleus may further improve rehabilitation in these patients who would have been deaf some years ago.

Keywords: Rehabilitation; hearing functions; neurofibromatosis type 2.

Introduction

This report will focus on some recent developments concerning an artificial sense. Building an artificial sense is one of the many efforts in Functional Neurosurgery and Neuromodulation, where the close collaboration between computer scientists, basic scientists and clinicians has been very successful. The most remarkable progress in this field has been made in constructing the artificial sense of hearing- the "bionic ear". Today many formerly deaf individuals with auditory implants are able to talk on the telephone with relative ease.

The normal ear is a device that transforms mechanical stimuli into electrical impulses. Low frequencies for examples cause a movement at the end of the basilar membrane and the information is transformed here into impulses of the cochlear nerve. The cochlear nerve transmits this information to the dorsal and ventral cochlear nucleus and to other ascending pathways like the nuclei of the superior olive, the lateral lemniscus and finally: to the auditory cortex.

With a hearing aid, we have access to the auditory system at three different locations:

Most patients with reduced hearing may be helped with a conventional hearing aid that basically amplifies the acoustic information and gives the amplified signal to the external ear. If damage of the middle or inner ear is the cause of hearing loss, then a cochlear implant can help in severe or total bilateral hearing

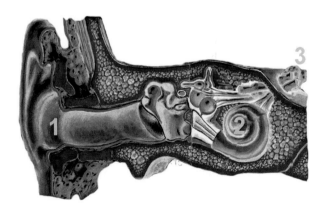

Fig. 1. (*1*) On the natural way through the external ear (Conventional hearing aid). (*2*) Through the cochlea in the case of a lesion of the inner ear (Cochlear implant). (*3*) At the level of the cochlear nucleus (Auditory brainstem implant, ABI)

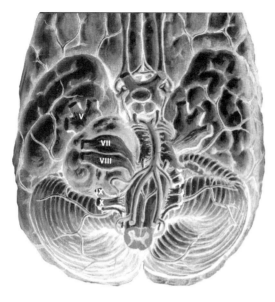

Fig. 2. Tumour at the 8th cranial nerve compressing the cranial nerves 5, 7, 8, 9, 10 and the brainstem

loss. But if the 8th nerve is damaged, then a cochlear implant is not useful. In these cases the only means of recovery is the electrical stimulation of the cochlear nucleus in the brainstem through an auditory implant (ABI).

Who needs an ABI? Individuals with Neurofibromatosis 2, in short: NF2 are a good indication. NF2 is characterized by tumours of the central nervous system, particularly the eigth cranial nerves. NF2 is a genetic disease that is passed from parent to a child at the time of conception and affects about 1 in 40000 people without regard to sex or race. However about 50% are spontaneous new mutations. Only a couple of years ago the exact location was identified on chromosome 22. Almost all individuals with NF2 develop tumours of the 8th cranial nerves.

Therapy may be conservative and "wait and see" in small tumours, but in most cases a microsurgical operation is needed to prevent further tumour growth. Due to the size and location of the tumours, deafness is a very frequent complication, either by destruction of the auditory nerve due to the tumour itself, or as a complication of the operation. Cochlear implants are only sometimes useful for these patients because during tumour removal usually the 8th nerve cannot be preserved especially in large tumours. Until some years ago, lip-reading and sign language had been the only communication modes available to these patients. For these patients, an auditory brainstem implant is ap-

propriate. The first ABI device was developed at the House Ear Institute, Los Angeles in 1979.

What are the components of an auditory brainstem implant? There are internal and external components. Most important is the stimulating electrode. Modern electrodes are multipolar; they are designed as an array of up to 20 electrodes, which are placed on Teflon felt to keep them in place at the implanted location. The electrodes are placed in the lateral recess of the fourth ventricle, next to the cochlear nuclei. The implanted electrodes stimulate circumscribed groups of neurons in the cochlear nucleus. The information is separated into different frequency bands; these are assigned to different electrodes.

Correct electrode placement depends on accurate identification of anatomic landmarks and on intrasurgical electrophysiologic monitoring. Electrically evoked auditory brain stem responses obtained by stimulation through the electrode array are monitored as well as electromyographic activity from cranial nerves 7 and 9 to reduce the risk of side effects. The electrode is connected to a receiver device which has a ground wire fixed at the temporal bone. The external components have changed a lot. Earlier systems were little computers with long cables and heavy batteries like big Walkman. Modern systems are mostly "behind the ear" systems. They are becoming smaller with every generation. Another aspect of the implanted components is important for follow-up examinations: It is possible to perform an MRI examination for follow up. Possible tumour growth of the contralateral side can be assessed by MRI without significant artefacts and without danger to the patient.

The Cologne/Würzburg ABI project was initiated in 1997. 12 ABI systems were implanted in 11 patients. One patient had to be reoperated because of postoperative dislocation of the electrode. 10 patients are using the ABI with benefit; the results of the Cologne/Würzburg ABI project are displayed in Table 1.

In all but one patient tonotopy could be demonstrated. Sound recognition, sound discrimination and speech recognition could also be demonstrated in all but one patient [6]. When lip-reading alone is compared to lip-reading with the ABI, sentence recognition improved about 30% on average with the auditory brainstem implant. Patient No 8 for example had a number recognition score of 65% with the implant alone. When the ABI was used together with lip reading, number recognition was 100%. The best patient scores 96% IS and 41% MS (ABI only). After ABI im-

Table 1. *CIS-ABI: Audiological Results of the Cologne/Würzburg ABI Project*

Patient nr.	Tonotopy	Sound recogn.	Sound discr.	Speech recogn.	IS LR/ R+ ABI	FN/MS ABI
1	+	+	+	+	n.i.	contralat. hearing
2	+	+	+	+	32–61%	n.i.
3	+	+	+	+	19–57%	45% MS
4	+	+	+	+	65(A)–96%	95%/41%
5	+	+	+	+	43–71%	45%/10%
6	–	–	–	–	n.i.	non-user
7	+	+	+	+	n.i.	hearing
8	+	+	+	+	50–76%	65% ABI/–100% LR + ABI
9	+	+	+	+	25% ABI	95% CS
10	+	+	+	+	n.i.	1. fitting
11	+	+	+	+	17–51%	1. fitting

n.i. Not investigated; *IS* Innsbruck Sentences; *FN* Freiburg Numbers; *MS* Monosyllables; *LR* Lip reading; *CS* Closed set; *A* ABI only.

plantation she was able to communicate independently and to use the telephone.

Conclusions

The auditory brainstem implant (ABI) is the only possibility for hearing rehabilitation following surgical treatment of bilateral neurinomas with destruction of the auditory nerve. The development of the ABI has significantly reduced the communication handicap experienced by many individuals with NF2. The implant allows recovery of auditory sensation, recognition of environmental noises and help lip-reading.

A coordinated multidisciplinary team is essential for a successful ABI program. In the future new developments in the field of speech-processing strategies and new electrode design accessing the tonotopic organization of the cochlear nucleus will further improve ABI performance.

References

1. Otto SR, Shannon RV, Brackmann DE (1998) The multichannel auditory brainstem implant (ABI): results in 20 patients. Otolaryngol Head Neck Surg 118: 291–303
2. Shannon RV, Fayad J, Moore J, Lo W, O'Leary M, Otto S, Nelson R (1993) Auditory brainstem implant: 2. postsurgical issues and performance. Otolaryngol Head Neck Surg 108: 634–642
3. Staller S, Otto SR, Menapace SR (1995) Clinical trials of the auditory brainstem implant. Audio Today 7: 9–12

Correspondence: J. Kuchta, Department of Neurosurgery and Department of ENT-Surgery, University of Cologne, Cologne, Germany.

Acta Neurochir (2001) [Suppl] 79: 113–115
© Springer-Verlag 2001

Electrical Stimulation of the Sural Nerve Partially Compensates Effects of Central Fatigue

J. D. Rollnik and **R. Dengler**

Medical School of Hannover, Department of Neurology and Clinical Neurophysiology, Hannover, Germany

Summary

Objectives. Depression of motor evoked potentials (MEPs) following transcranial magnetic stimulation (TMS) may be a sign of central motor fatigue. Abnormal fatigue can be observed in MS patients. We have examined whether post-exercise MEP depression can be compensated by application of sensory stimuli prior to TMS.

Methods. We studied 15 healthy volunteers (aged 21 to 28 years) who were required to perform an exercise protocol of ankle dorsiflexion until force fell below 66% of maximum force. MEPs were recorded from the right tibialis anterior muscle. Prior to TMS, electrical stimuli were applied to the ipsilateral sural nerve with an individual interstimulus interval between 50 to 80 ms.

Results. MEP areas decreased after exercise. When a sensory stimulus was administered MEPs did not change.

Discussion. We conclude that the effects of central fatigue may be – at least partially compensated – by application of sensory stimuli. Sensory stimulation (e.g. by implantation of a neurostimulator) might be a useful therapy for abnormal central fatigue.

Keywords: Functional electrical stimulation; coma stimulation; central fatigue.

Introduction

Abnormal central motor fatigue poses a problem in neurorehabilitation and may occur in patients with lesions of the corticospinal system [6]. Fatigue of the motor system is characterized by a decrease of force generated by the neuromuscular system during sustained or repeated muscle activity. Central motor fatigue leads to a post-exercise depression of MEPs and results from reduced neural drive proximal to the anterior horn cell [6]. The origin of central fatigue is still a matter of discussion, but some authors suggested that the frontal cortex and basal ganglia might be involved [3]. MEPs may be facilitated by sensory stimulation prior to TMS [1]. Short-interval facilitation, which is supposed to be mediated through spinal mechanisms, takes place when a sensory stimulus is applied some 10 ms prior to TMS. Long-interval facilitation reaches its optimum between 30 and 50 ms for upper and 50 to 80 ms for lower limbs and is probably mediated through cortical neurons [2]. This paper presents results of a study with healthy volunteers [5].

Methods

We studied 15 healthy right-handed volunteers (9 men and 6 women), aged 21 to 28 years (mean 24.7, SD = 2.2). All subjects gave written informed consent to the experimental procedure. Subjects lay on a bed with hip flexed to 90°, the knee flexed to 90°, and the ankle at 100°. A strain gauge was attached to the right ankle and foot in order to perform force measurements of ankle dorsiflexion. Single electrical stimuli of the sural nerve were applied by surface electrodes placed at the lateral malleolus. Duration of the stimulus was 0.1 ms and the intensity was two times perception threshold. Using a D4030 Digitimer (Digitimer Ltd., Hertfordshire, UK), the conditioning sensory stimuli were given at individually determined interstimulus intervals (50 to 80 ms prior to TMS) that had produced MEPs with the largest areas in prior trials, i.e., the strongest facilitation. For this purpose, intervals between 40 and 100 ms were tested in random order and steps of 10 ms in each subject. The interval with the strongest MEP facilitation was used as the interstimulus interval throughout the experiment. During the experiment a sensory stimulus preceded TMS in 10 of 20 trials (in random order). Transcranial magnetic stimuli (MagStim 200; The MagStim Company Ltd., Whitland, UK) were applied over the vertex with a double-cone coil (current in the coil was directed anteriorly). MEPs were recorded from the right tibialis anterior and gastrocnemius muscles with surface EMG electrodes at rest. The intensity of TMS was set at 20% above the motor threshold (MT). Magnetic stimulation was followed immediately by supramaximal electrical stimuli (1 Hz) applied to the right peroneal nerve to evoke the M-wave and 10 F-waves in the right tibialis anterior muscle. The subjects had to perform an exercise protocol (dorsiflexion of the foot) at a level of 70% of baseline maximum force (6 seconds exercise, 4 seconds rest) until force fell below 66% of maximum force, which was set as endurance limit. Maximum force was determined as the strongest force from three consecutive trials with a duration of 1 second (prior to the experiment, at baseline).

Results

We found that maximum force was significantly reduced after exercise (Friedman-test: $\chi^2 = 18.24$, df = 3; p < 0.001; Fig. 1). Immediately after exercise, force was decreased to a mean of 69.9% (SD = 9.8) of pre-exercise values. 15 minutes after exercise maximum force increased to 90.8% (SD = 14.2), and 30 minutes after exercise to 93.3% (SD = 14.5) of baseline levels. The endurance limit was reached after a mean of 5.9 minutes (SD = 7.3; range 2.5–30 minutes). In the absence of sensory stimulation, areas of rectified MEPs from the tibialis anterior muscle decreased im-mediately after exercise (Fig. 2) to 88.2% (SD = 50.5), to 62.1% (SD = 33.7) after 15 min, and to 81.0% (SD = 64.0) after 30 min. This MEP area reduction was highly significant (Friedman-test: mean rank 3.50 before exercise, 2.58 immediately after exercise, 1.75 after 15 min, and 2.17 after 30 min; $\chi^2 = 12.10$, df = 3, p = 0.007). When an electrical stimulus preceded TMS (Fig. 2) areas of rectified MEPs did not change sig-nificantly (92.4% (SD = 44.8) immediately after exer-cise, 82.2% (SD = 32.9) after 15 min, and 95.2% (SD = 41.2) after 30 min; $\chi^2 = 1.84$, df = 3, n.s.). Comparing MEP areas with and without prior electri-cal stimulation (using Kruskal-Wallis-tests), we could

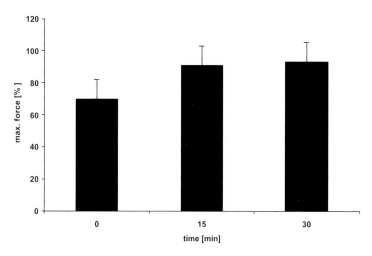

Fig. 1. Maximum force immediately after the exercise (0), 15 and 30 minutes post-exercise. Force values are expressed as percent of baseline maximum force (pre-exercise maximum force). Standard deviation is indicated on top of bars (Fig. modified from [4])

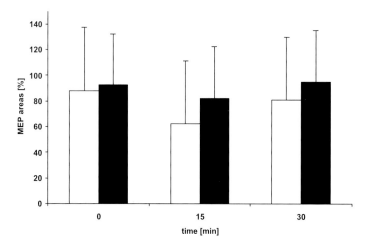

Fig. 2. Areas of rectified MEPs with and without conditioning electrical stimulation of the sural nerve. MEP area values are expressed as percent of pre-exercise values. Post-exercise there was a significant decrease of MEP areas when no sensory stimulation took place. No signif-icant changes could be observed when there was an electrical stimulus prior to TMS. Areas were significantly higher after 15 and 30 min when electrical stimulation was performed. Standard deviation is indicated on top of bars (Fig. modified from [4]) □ without, ■ with

not find significant differences at baseline ($\chi^2 = 1.47$, df $= 1$, n.s.) and immediately after exercise ($\chi^2 = 2.95$, df $= 1$, p $= 0.086$), but 15 min ($\chi^2 = 4.05$, df $= 1$, p $= 0.044$) and 30 min ($\chi^2 = 5.22$, df $= 1$, p $= 0.022$) later, MEP areas were significantly higher with conditioning sural stimulation. M- and F-waves, TMCT and CMCT did not change before and after exercise. Oral body temperature pre- and post-exercise did not change. We could not find significant MEP changes induced by exercise or by electrical stimulation in the antagonist muscle (gastrocnemius muscle), either.

Discussion

After an exhausting exercise, central fatigue may occur leading to post-exercise MEP depression without M-wave changes [6]. It is well known that sensory stimuli may facilitate MEPs [1]. This MEP facilitation follows sensory stimulation at short and long intervals. Short-interval facilitation is believed to arise on a spinal level, whereas long-interval facilitation is probably mediated through cortical mechanisms. We found that sensory stimuli elevated previously depressed MEPs (when central fatigue is assumed).

The site of this effect cannot be determined easily. The results of our study indicate that it is not the neuromuscular junction (unchanged M-responses). The fact that the latencies used were within range of long-interval facilitation suggests that cortical mechanisms may be involved. The processing of facilitation and fatigue might take place in these neurons. In addition, the dorsolateral prefrontal cortex (DLPFC) is essential in central motor control [4]. In a previous study, we demonstrated that activation of DLPFC using rapid-rate repetitive TMS (rTMS) may induce MEP depression [4]. This finding reflects that the DLPFC is able to reduce motor cortex excitability. Further, sensory information might be transmitted to frontal areas and thus reduces its inhibiting influence. In addition, there are a few observations that the frontal cortex plays a crucial role in the phenomenon of central fatigue. Roelcke *et al.* [3] demonstrated a reduced glucose metabolism in the frontal cortex and basal ganglia of MS patients with fatigue.

In summary, we could demonstrate that sensory input may partially compensate fatigue-induced MEP depression. There are good reasons to believe that this mechanism could be mediated through a transcortical loop involving frontal cortical areas. Further studies on this topic, combining neurophysiological methods with functional imaging, are strongly encouraged. The results of the study might point to therapies of abnormal central fatigue in the near future:

(1) One target of future therapies could be the peripheral nerve system. As demonstrated with the present study, sensory stimulation might be able to compensate effects of central fatigue [5]. Therefore, a neurostimulator could be implanted to stimulate sensory nerve fibers of limbs involved.

(2) The other target to treat abnormal central fatigue might be the prefrontal cortex. rTMS of the prefrontal system [4] might interfere with central structures involved in motor fatigue. Thus, rTMS could be a useful tool in neurorehabilitation.

References

1. Dengler R, Schubert M, Wohlfarth K, Czapowski D (1995) An approach to study the role of the corticospinal tract in central fatigue. Electroencephalogr Clin Neurophysiol 97: S58
2. Nielsen J, Petersen N, Fedirchuk B (1997) Evidence suggesting a transcortical pathway from cutaneous foot afferents to tibialis anterior motoneurones in man. J Physiol 473–484
3. Roelcke U, Kappos L, Lechner-Scott J, Brunnschweiler H, Huber S, Ammann W, Plohmann A, Dellas S, Maguire RP, Missimer J, Radu EW, Steck A, Leenders KL (1997) Reduced glucose metabolism in the frontal cortex and basal ganglia of multiple sclerosis patients with fatigue: a 18F-flurodeoxyglucose positron emission tomography study. Neurology 48(6): 1566–1571
4. Rollnik JD, Schubert M, Dengler R (2000) Subthreshold prefrontal repetitive transcranial magnetic stimulation reduces motor cortex excitability. Muscle Nerve 23(1): 112–114
5. Rollnik JD, Schubert M, Albrecht J, Wohlfarth K, Dengler R (2000) Effects of somatosensory input on central fatigue: a pilot study. Clin Neurophysiol (in press)
6. Schubert M, Wohlfarth K, Rollnik JD, Dengler R (1998) Walking and fatigue in multiple sclerosis: The role of the corticospinal system. Muscle Nerve 21: 1068–1070

Correspondence: J. D. Rollnik, Medical School of Hannover, Department of Neurology and Clinical Neurophysiology, Hannover, Germany.

Acta Neurochir (2001) [Suppl] 79: 117–122

Management of Upper and Lower Limb Spasticity in Neuro-Rehabilitation

S. Hesse, C. Werner, A. Bardeleben, and **B. Brandl-Hesse**

Klinik Berlin Department of Neurological Rehabilitation, Free University Berlin, Germany

Summary

This article reviews the treatment of upper and lower limb spasticity in neurological rehabilitation. Botulinum toxin A proved effective in several placebo-controlled studies reducing muscle tone, easing hand hygiene and nursing, improving upper limb motor functions and gait ability. The effects are reversible and the toxin is well tolerated. Electrical stimulation, tonic stretch post injection and the active use of the treated extremity are means to increase the effectiveness of the costly therapy. Phenol 5% is an alternative in case of budget constraints, but the technique is demanding and side effects are more frequent. Further, task-specific repetitive therapy should follow the successful treatment of focal spasticity in eligible patients to get the maximum profit with regard to disability.

Keywords: Botulinum toxin; spasticity; task-specific therapy.

Introduction

In neurorehabilitation spasticity is more than the treatment of enhanced stretch reflexes. Patients do not suffer from exaggerated reflexes but from impaired function due to a spastic deformity. In stroke patients this shows either as a flexor pattern of the upper extremity or as an equinovarus deformity of the feet. Patients cannot use their hands, hand hygiene or dressing are impaired. With regard to gait, patients cannot clear the ground during the swing phase, hit the ground with the forefoot instead of the heel, improperly load their limb, and may suffer from a sprained ankle.

Up until the 1990s, physical treatment regimes (e.g. physiotherapy, casting, electrical stimulation, cycling, tendon transfer etc.) and oral antispastic medications were the only therapeutic options for the management of spasticity. The effects, however, were either of short duration, could result in a functional deterioration caused by general weakness or were non-reversible, as is the case with surgical operations. Since then, Botulinum toxin A (BTX) which was established in the treatment of dystonia, evolved as a new and promising alternative in the management of spasticity [4]. The basic aim is to weaken the muscles responsible for the spastic deformity selectively. BTX effects a local paresis, the reversible effects start approximately one week after the injection and last 3 to 4 months. Most of the patients tolerate the toxin well. Minor, reversible side effects were disabling weakness of injected and non-injected muscles, a temporary bladder paresis, and a mild dysphagia after the treatment of adductor spasticity.

This review will discuss articles on the BTX treatment of adult upper and lower limb spasticity, address questions concerning treatment technique and subsequent functional training programs.7

Botulinum Toxin A Treatment of Adult Upper Limb Flexor Spasticity

Following several open studies, Simpson *et al.* [19] were the first to report a randomised, double-blind, placebo-controlled trial using BtxA in 39 individuals with spastic upper extremities. The authors injected electromyogram (EMG)-guided placebo or a total dosage of 75, 150 and 300 units of the US-product into three muscles: Biceps brachii (4 injection sites, 65% of total dosage), flexor carpi radialis (one site, 25% of total dosage) and ulnaris (one site, 15% of total dosage). Only the treatment with the highest dose resulted in a statistically significant mean decrease of muscle tone at 2, 4 and 6 weeks after injection. There were no adverse reactions. No significant differences were found between placebo and treatment groups for motor functions of the affected upper extremity, pain, care-giver dependency and competence in daily activities. A recent placebo-controlled study with 82 stroke patients investigated the effect of 500, 1000 and 1500 units Dysport for the treatment of upper limb spasticity. It revealed a significant muscle tone reduction for all three dosages as compared to placebo, competence in daily activities and motor functions however did not differ among groups [2]. The authors injected the toxin or placebo into five muscles of the affected arm.

The results of these two controlled studies are not fully in accord with open studies [15, 16, 21] which reported an increased range of motion, a reduction in pain, a facilitation of hand hygiene and an improved motor function of the extensor muscles after BtxA treatment with considerably less toxin. Reiter and co-workers [16], for instance, described an improved hand function after injection in those patients who exhibited a residual voluntary activation of their paretic finger extensors. Plegic patients, however, did not profit from the injection with regard to their motor function. Recently, one group reported the injection of the Mm. lumbricales in case of a persistent flexor deformity of the fingers following a first injection of the long finger flexors in the forearm [14]. Repeated botulinum toxin injection over a period of 3 years effected an unchanging effectiveness in the management of focal upper limb spasticity after stroke [12].

Botulinum Toxin A Treatment of Adult Lower Limb Spasticity

Our group was among the first to show the beneficial effect of BTX in the treatment of equinovarus deformity after stroke [9]. Following the injection of the plantar flexors patients improved their mode of initial contact, advanced their bodies more well, (Fig. 1) and walked faster. This finding was confirmed by a subsequent placebo-controlled study by Burbaud *et al.* [3]. The authors injected EMG-guided placebo or a total dosage of 1000 units of the UK product into the muscles soleus, gastrocnemius, tibialis posterior and flexor digitorum longus. Patients reported a clear subjective improvement in foot spasticity after BtxA, but not after placebo administration. Significant changes were noted in Ashworth scale values for ankle extensor and invertors, and for active ankle dorsiflexion up to three months after injection. Gait velocity was improved slightly but not significantly after the injection of BtxA. The authors further reported that BtxA was less effective in patients with longer duration of spasticity.

The fact that patients could actively dorsiflex their ankles after the injection might be explained by a reduced reciprocal inhibition via the Ia extensor afferents which inhibits flexor motor neurones in spastic lower limbs [1]. In confirmation, one study in mice [18] showed that BtxA not only effected extrafusal but

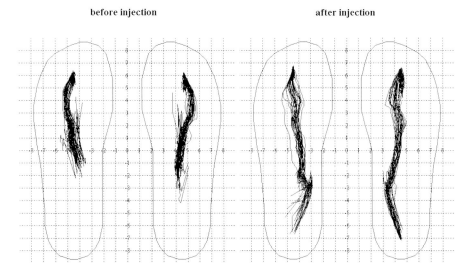

before injection   after injection

Fig. 1. Trajectories of the force point of action in a right hemiparetic patient before and two weeks after the injection of botulinum toxin A

before injection

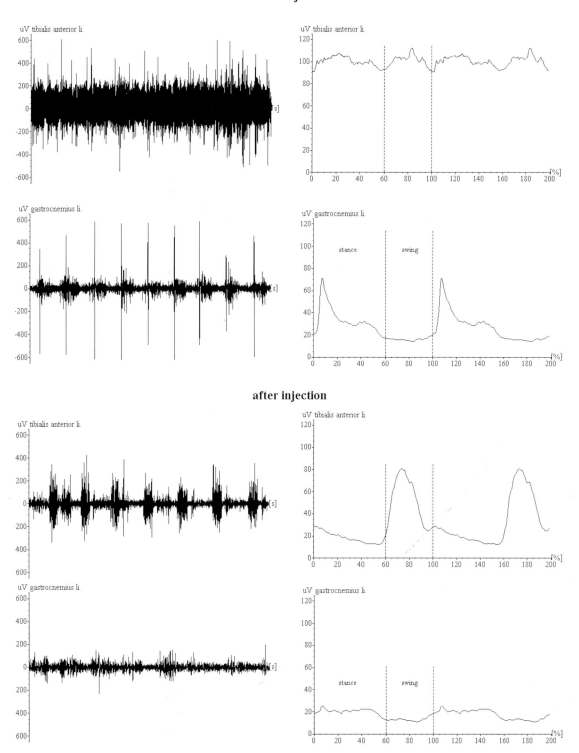

after injection

Fig. 2. Averaged and normalised electromyogram of the gastrocnemius and tibialis anterior muscles of a diplegic child before (above) and after (below) treatment with Botulinum toxin of the gastrocnemius muscle. Note the corrected activation pattern of the non-injected tibialis anterior muscle

also cholinergically enervated intrafusal muscle fibers, thereby reducing the spindle afferent discharge. A direct effect on the enervating motor neurones (e.g. by a retrograde axonal transport) could not be documented in cats with therapeutically common dosages [13].

Ankle muscle activity during gait was assessed in stroke patients with a spastic drop foot before and after the injection of 400 units of the US product into the plantar flexors [6]. Preferentially, the toxin diminished the stretch-related premature activity, whereas the functional activity of the plantar flexors at midstance was less affected. The presence of premature activity of the plantar flexors correlated with a good therapeutic effect. On the other hand, a very low EMG activity level (indicating altered mechanical properties) predicted a poor result, confirming the necessity to exclude partial muscle contracture as much as possible before injection. Subsequent dynamic EMG recordings further helped to select the best muscles for injection following the slogan: the more muscle activity and the more disturbed the motor pattern, the better are the results. Seldom, the tibialis anterior of hemiparetic subjects shows a high tonic activation pattern, then adding to impairing foot inversion due to its medial insertion. In these cases, its injection with BTX is recommended. Other potential "candidates" are the soleus muscle and the tibialis posterior. Both gastrocnemius heads, on the other hand, often show a low activity; correspondingly an exclusive injection of the gastrocnemius muscles with a neurolytic agent will not help much.

Another interesting aspect of the BTX injection of the plantar flexors (a mean of 23 units Dysport/kg body weight), particularly in CP children, is a corrected pattern of the (non-injected) antagonistic tibialis anterior muscle being transformed from a tonic into a phasic timely correct mode [5], (Fig. 2). Possible explanation is the above mentioned reduced reciprocal inhibition of the flexor muscle following the now recognised action of BTX on the intrafusal muscle fibres altering the Ia-afferents.

In MS patients suffering from disabling adductor spasticity two placebo-controlled studies were reported. Snow and co-workers found that the injection of a total dosage of 400 units of Botox into both adductor muscles significantly reduced the muscle tone and eased hygiene as compared to placebo [20]. More recently, a multi-centre trial confirmed these results with an injection of 1500 units Dysport into both adductor muscle groups [11].

Technical Aspects

Despite proper muscle selection and EMG-guided injection technique the results of BTX treatment of spasticity did not match the results of dystonic muscles. Early animal literature helped to understand this difference. Hughes and Walker [10] had used the N. phrenicus-diaphragm preparation of the rat and showed elegantly that the activity of the terminal nerve ends and the uptake and efficacy of BTX correlated with each other. Furthermore, an external stimulation of the N. phrenicus increased the uptake of the toxin. Dystonic muscles are highly active whereas spastic muscles exhibit a low activity. Paresis adds to the little activity level of terminal nerve ends in spastic muscles. To increase the effectiveness of the costly BTX injection one should therefore encourage patients to use their extremities after treatment vigorously. For patients who are unable to use their extremities our group introduced two-channel electrical stimulation of the antagonistic and agonistic muscles immediately after the treatment. The current protocol recommends a 30-min stimulation (25 Hz, 0.25 ms pulse width, and intensity above motor threshold to elicit a minimal joint movement) five times a day for three days following the injection. The additional stimulation of the antagonistic muscle (for instance of the wrist extensors) serves two purposes: the spasticity-related flexor deformity is corrected, and eliciting a stretch reflex further enhances the activity level of the spastic flexor muscles. A double-blind placebo-controlled study [7] in hemiparetic subjects suffering from an upper limb flexor spasticity confirmed this technique's value: the group receiving verum (1000 units Dysport) plus stimulation profited most with regard to spasticity reduction and better hand hygiene as compared to the other three groups receiving either placebo with and without stimulation or the verum alone.

Another established clinical technique to increase the effectiveness of the BTX-treatment is a subsequent tonic stretch of the affected extremity. As mentioned above, a chronic spastic deformity is not only neurogenic but also results from concomitant changes of the muscle's mechanical properties. As the neurolytic agent BTX only addresses the neurogenic component, a consequent tonic stretch of the shortened muscle should also help to correct the deformity. In the treatment of the upper extremity we recommend an upholstered and mouldable splint – alternatives are thermoplastic splints, serial castings or taping. For taping,

Reiter and co-workers investigated stroke patients suffering from a spastic drop foot [17]. Two groups of patients were investigated. One group was injected with a high dose of toxin while the other group received a lower dose of BTX in combination with ankle taping for three weeks. Both groups experienced a comparable muscle tone reduction and an improvement of ground level walking velocity. Consequently, one should apply a tonic stretch of the injected muscles for at least three weeks.

Further means to increase the effectiveness of the toxin are a higher dilution volume according to clinical experience. In the early nineties dilutions of 1.0–2.5 ml/vial were common; nowadays several groups use volumes up to 10 ml/vial to enhance the diffusion of the toxin within the muscle.

With regard to the injection technique, EMG-guidance is recommended in deep muscles, for instance in the region of the forearm. The monopolar needles can be connected to a stimulator, a visible muscle twitch at a minimal stimulation intensity (< 5 mA) indicates the vicinity of the motor point and a good injection site. The number of injection sites is debatable. In large volume muscles with a scattered profile of the nerve entry zone in the muscle several sites are recommended. To exclude a contracture and thus a negative result after BTX injection, one can set up a nerve block, for instance of the N. tibialis with 5–8 ml Bupivacain 0.5%.

Despite any means to save toxin, budget constraints may limit the use of Botulinum toxin. The alternative is phenol 5%. Good indications are a severe elbow flexor spasticity (N. musculocutaneus), and a spastic drop foot (N. tibialis). EMG- and stimulator-guidance is mandatory to find the optimal injection site. One should only administer phenol 5% when a stimulation intensity of less than 3 mA causes a visible muscle twitch. In comparison to BTX, the injection technique of Phenol is more demanding, and side effects (pain, inflammation and dysaesthesia) are more likely to occur. On the other hand, phenol causes an immediate effect which can last up to eight months.

Task-Specific Repetitive Therapy

Successful focal treatment of spasticity may open a window for functional therapy. For instance, the correction of a spastic drop foot should be followed by gait therapy to obtain the maximum profit. Most promising is a task-specific repetitive approach, i.e. who wants to relearn walking has to walk. To enable wheelchair-bound subjects the practise of complex gait cycles without overstraining therapists, an electro-mechanical gait trainer was designed [8], (Fig. 3). The harness-secured patient is positioned on two foot plates whose movements simulate stance and swing in a highly symmetric manner with a physiological ratio of 60% to 40% between stance and swing. A velocity-controlled motor drive supports the patient according to his abilities, and the movement of the CoM is controlled in vertical and horizontal direction. During a net walking time of 20 min a patient practises about 1200 step cycles. Recent

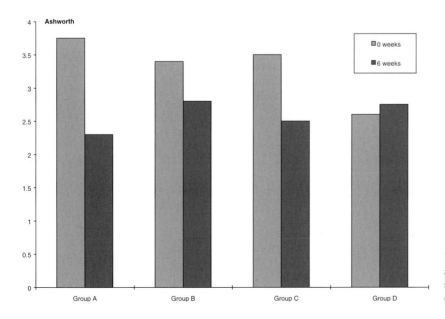

Fig. 3. Electro-mechanical gait trainer enabling the repetitive practise of a highly symmetric gait-like movement without overstraining therapists

clinical trials showed that chronic hemiparetic patients can improve their gait ability even years after stroke-onset. Currently, several clinical trials are on the way to further elucidate the effectiveness of the device.

In conclusion, BTX is becoming an effective and well established treatment option of spasticity after stroke. Electrical stimulation and tonic stretch following the injection may help to increase the effectiveness of the costly treatment. Phenol 5% is an alternative in case of budget constraints. Further, task-specific repetitive therapy should be following the successful treatment of focal spasticity.

References

1. Artieda J, Quesada P, Obeso JA (1991) Reciprocal Ia inhibition in spastic hemiplegia. Neurology 41: 286–289
2. Bakheit AM, Thilmann AF, Ward AB, Poewe W, Wissel J, Muller J, Benecke R, Collin C, Muller F, Ward CD, Neumann C (2000) A randomized, double-blind, placebo-controlled, dose-ranging study to compare the efficacy and safety of three doses of Botulinum toxin type A (Dysport) with placebo in upper limb spasticity after stroke. Stroke 31: 2402–2406
3. Burbaud P, Wiart L, Dubos JL, Gaujard E, Debeillex X, Joseph PA, Mazaux JM, Bioulac B, Barat M, Lagueny A (1996) A randomised, double blind, placebo controlled trial of botulinum toxin in the treatment of spastic foot in hemiparetic patients. J Neurol Neurosurg Psychiatry 61: 265–269
4. Das TK, Park DM (1989) Botulinum toxin in treating spasticity. Br J Clin Pharmacol 43: 401–402
5. Hesse S, Brandl-Hesse B, Seidel U, Doll B, Gregoric M (2000) Lower limb muscle activity in ambulatory children with cerebral palsy before and after the treatment with Botulinum toxin A. Restorative Neurology and Neuroscience 15: 1–8
6. Hesse S, Krajnik J, Lücke D, Jahnke MT, Gregoric M, Mauritz KH (1996) Ankle muscle activity before and after botulinum toxin therapy for lower limb extensor spasticity in chronic hemiparetic patients: Stroke 27: 455–460
7. Hesse S, Reiter F, Konrad M, Uhlenbrock D, Jahnke MT (1998) Botulinum toxin type A and short-term electrical stimulation in the treatment of upper limb flexor spasticity after stroke: a randomised, double-blind, placebo-controlled trial. Clin Rehab 12: 381
8. Hesse S, Uhlenbrock D, Werner C, Bardeleben A (2000) A mechanized gait trainer for restoring gait in non-ambulatory subjects. Arch Phys Med Rehab 81: 1158–1162
9. Hesse S, Lücke D, Malezic M, Bertelt C, Friedrich H, Mauritz KH (1994) Botulinum toxin therapy for lower limb extensor spasticity. J Neurol Neurosurg Psychiatry 57: 1321–1325
10. Hughes R, Walker BC (1962) Influence of nerve-ending activity and of drugs on the rate of paralysis of rat diaphragm preparations by Clostridium botulinum type toxin A. J Physiol 160: 221–233
11. Hyman N, Branes M, Bhakta B, Cozens A, Bakheit M, Kreczy-Kleedorfer B, Poewe W, Wissel J, Bain B, Glickman S, Sayer A, Richardson A, Dott C (2000) Botulinum toxin (Dysport) treatment of hip adductor spasticity in multiple sclerosis: a prosepctive, randomised, double blind, placebo controlled, dose ranging study. J Neurol Neurosurg Psychiatry 68: 707–712
12. Lagalla G, Danni M, Reiter F, Ceravolo MG, Provinciali L (2000) Post-stroke spasticity management with repeated Botulinum toxin injections in the upper limb. Am J Phys Med Rehab 79: 377–384
13. Moreno-Lopez B, Pastor AM, de la Cruz RR, Delgado-Garcia JM (1997) Dose-dependent central effects of botulinum neuro-toxin type A: a pilot study in the alert behaving cat. Neurology 48: 456–464
14. Palmer DT, Horn LJ, Harmon RL (1998) Botulinumtoxin treatment of lumbrical spasticity. Am J Phys Med Rehab 77: 349–350
15. Pierson SH, Katz DI, Tarsy D (1996) Botulinum toxin A in the treatment of spasticity: functional implications in patient selection. Arch Phys Med Rehab 77: 717–721
16. Reiter F, Danni M, Ceravolo MG, Provinciali L (1996) Disability changes after treatment of upper limb spasticity with botulinum toxin. J Neurol Rehab 10: 47–52
17. Reiter F, Danni M, Lagalla G, Ceravolo G, Provinciali L (1998) Low-dose botulinum toxin with ankle taping for the treatment of spastic equinovarus foot after stroke. Arch Phys Med Rehab 79: 532–535
18. Rosales RL, Arimura K, Takenaga S, Osame M (1996) Extrafusal and intrafusal muscle effects in experimental botulinum toxin-A injection. Muscle Nerve 19: 488–496
19. Simpson DM, Alexander DN, O'Brian CF, Tagliati M, Aswad AS, Leon JM, Gibson J, Mordaund JM, Monaghan EP (1996) Botulinum toxin type A in the treatment of upper extremity spasticity: a randomized, double-blind, placebo-controlled trial. Neurology 46: 1306–1310
20. Snow BJ, Tsui JKC, Bhatt MH, Varelas M, Hashimoto SA, Calne DB (1990) Treatment of spasticity with botulinum toxin: a double blind study. Ann Neurol 28: 512–515
21. Yablon SA, Benjamin TA, Ivanhoe CB, Boake C (1996) Botulinum toxin in severe upper extremity spasticity among patients with traumatic brain injury: an open-labeled trial. Neurology 47: 939–944

Correspondence: Stefan Hesse, M.D., Klinik Berlin, Department of Neurological Rehabilitation, Kladower Damm 223, 14089 Berlin, Germany.

Acta Neurochir (2001) [Suppl] 79: 123–126

Botulinum Toxin (DYSPORT) in Tension-Type Headaches

J. D. Rollnik and **R. Dengler**

Medical School of Hannover, Department of Neurology and Clinical Neurophysiology, Hannover, Germany

Summary

Objectives. Botulinum toxin type A is effective in the reduction of muscle tenderness and pain in many diseases associated with myofascial pain. Since increased muscle tension may contribute to tension-type headaches, injections of botulinum toxin could be of therapeutic value.

Methods/Patients. Results of own investigations are presented, in particular a double-blind, placebo-controlled study with 21 patients fulfilling the International Headache Society criteria for tension-type hedaches. Participants were randomly assigned to verum (pericranial injection of 10×20 MU DYSPORT) or placebo condition (injection of isotonic saline in the same manner).

Results. After 4, 8, and 12 weeks no significant differences between placebo and verum could be observed. Nevertheless, both groups significantly improved.

Discussion. The findings strongly suggest that higher doses or other injection sites might be necessary to achieve therapeutic effects of botulinum toxin in tension-type headaches. Actually, we are participating in a multi-center study using 500 MU of DYSPORT. Besides dose-finding problems, another explanation could be that peripheral mechanisms – such as increased pericranial muscle tension – only play a minor role in the pathogenesis of tension-type headaches.

Keywords: Botulinum toxin; headache.

Introduction

The clinical, epidemiologic, and societal impact of tension-type headache (TTH) is immense. It poses a problem in neurological rehabilitation, e.g. after head injuries. Chronic post-traumatic headaches have no special features, but are symptomatically identical to chronic tension-type headache [4]. The lifetime prevalence of TTH is up to 30% in a general population [3]. The clinical symptoms are consisting of ache or sensations of tightness, pressure, or constriction, widely varied in intensity, frequency, and duration [7]. The International Headache Society classification [5] excludes typical symptoms of migraine, and differentiates between episodic and chronic (more than 180 days per year) tension-type headache. The pathophysiology is complex but increased pericranial muscle tension may contribute to the development of tension headaches at least in a fraction of patients [7].

Botulinum toxin type A is a potent drug in the treatment of several diseases associated with inreased muscle tone, such as dystonia, facial hemispasm, spasticity, and unvoluntary co-contractions [9]. Botulinum toxin has also been found useful in the treatment of painful muscle spasms and myofascial pain syndrome [1, 2]. Some studies suggested that botulinum toxin could be of therapeutic value in tension-type-headache as well [8, 11, 12]. However, the results of these studies are conflicting. Zwart and colleagues [12] could not find any significant reduction in pain intensity nor in pressure pain threshold in six patients with tension headache (injection site: temporal muscles; dose: up to 30–40 MU BOTOX; Allergan, Irvine, Ca., USA). In contrast, Relja [8] treated ten patients in an open-label trial and reported positive effects (injection site: tender pericranial muscles; dose: 15–35 MU BOTOX). Wheeler [11] also described favourable effects in four cases (injection site: tender pericranial and neck muscles; dose: up to 160 MU BOTOX). A problem with these studies [8, 11, 12] is the small sample size and an open-label design. For this reason, we performed a double-blind placebo-controlled study on the efficacy of botulinum toxin type A (DYSPORT) in the treatment of patients with episodic and chronic tension-type headaches [10].

Patients and Methods

Patients

We enrolled 21 patients (mean age 37.4 years, SD = 14.3, range 19–63 years) with episodic and chronic tension-type headaches according to the International Headache Society classification. Exclusion criteria were anticoagulation, myasthenia gravis, pregnancy, breastfeeding period, predominantly operating factors (e.g. secondary gain, compensation, disability, and psychosocial factors), rebound analgesic headache syndrome, and symptomatic or other concomitant headaches. All participants presented with a normal magnetic resonance imaging (MRI) or computertomography of the head and were resistant to previous medication (including antidepressants). Concomitant medication was allowed (including analgesics and rescue medications) but patients were required to document carefully any pharamacotherapeutics in their home diary. In a double-blind placebo-controlled design, subjects were randomly assigned to placebo or verum condition. Both groups did not significantly differ with respect to sociodemographic data. There was a preponderance of episodic tension-type headache in both groups (9 in the placebo and 7 in the verum group; $\chi^2 = 2.0$; p = 0.16). The patients gave written informed consent to participate in the study, as required by the local ethics committee.

Outcome Parameters

The patients were carefully examined and then followed-up after 4, 8, and 12 weeks. Patients were asked to keep a home diary throughout the study (starting 4 weeks prior to the study) recording daily consumption of analgesics, pain intensity (visual analogue scale: range 0–10; 0 = no pain, 10 = strongest pain), site, and duration of headache attacks. Furthermore, patients were required to give a rating on the visual analogue scale (VAS).

Measurement of Muscle Tenderness

In addition, muscle tenderness was determined measuring the total tenderness score (TTS) and pressure pain threshold (PPT) [6] at baseline and during the follow-ups.

In a fraction of patients, EMG surface activity was measured in order to evaluate muscle tension [6]. Frontal and anterior temporal muscles on both sides were examined. The electrodes on the temporal muscles were placed 2 cm behind the lateral eye margin and 2 cm above the orbito-meatal line. The frontal muscles were studied with the electrodes 2 cm above the superior orbital margin. Figure 1 illustrates EMG recordings: (A) shows surface EMG of a TTH patient without headache, (B) of a subject with headache during recording. Apparently, EMG activity at rest was more accentuated in the patient with headaches.

Botulinum Toxin Injections

Injections were given into the pericranial muscles circular around the head (2 injections into the frontooccipital muscle and 3 into the temporal muscles bilaterally, according to 10/20 system: Fp1/Fp2, F7/F8, T3/T4, T5/T6, O1/O2, Fig. 2). Verum treatment was carried out with 20 MU DYSPORT (Speywood Ltd., Wrexam, UK) per spot, diluted to 200 MU/ml (total dose: 10 × 20 MU = 200 MU/patient). Placebo was administered with 0.1 ml isotonic saline per injection site, given at the same spots as the botulinum toxin injections.

Results

At baseline (prior to injections), placebo and verum group did not differ significantly with respect to VAS. During the study, VAS values decreased for the whole group (paired difference for the 1st follow up: −1.04 (SD = 2.30), p = 0.051; 2nd follow-up −1.22 (SD = 2.86), p = 0.064; 3rd follow-up: −1.01 (SD = 2.37), p = 0.072), but no significant differences between placebo and verum treatment could be found (Fig. 3).

In addition, no significant differences between the treatment groups could be found as far as PPT, TTS, headache frequency, and consumption of analgesics are concerned.

Discussion

Increased pericranial muscle tension and tenderness may contribute to the development of tension headaches at least in some patients, but the pathogenesis has not been fully established yet [7]. Some authors believe that increased muscle tenderness only plays a minor role and that the underlying mechanism might be a central one. Beneficial effects of antidepressants also suggest a central origin.

The most important result of our study was that the whole group improved on the VAS, but we could not find any significant difference between placebo and verum treatment. This finding underlines that placebo-effects may be considerable, especially in headache studies. Therefore, some of the reported beneficial effects of botulinum toxin therapy might be due to this phenomenon. Needling and injections of saline or local anesthetics into muscle tender points have been reported helpful by removing nociceptive impulses. This mechanism could explain the overall improvement in our sample. The negative results of our study are in line with those of Zwart and co-workers [12] supporting the hypothesis that muscular tension only plays a minor role in the pathogenesis of tension-type headache. Nevertheless, EMG surface recordings indicated that pericranial muscles were more tense during headache attacks. On the basis of our findings [10], one might come to the conclusion that this increased muscular tension is secondary.

Another explanation of the negative findings of our study could be a dose-finding problem. We are now participating in a multi-center study using 500 MU DYSPORT. In addition, other muscle groups, in particular neck muscles, should be treated.

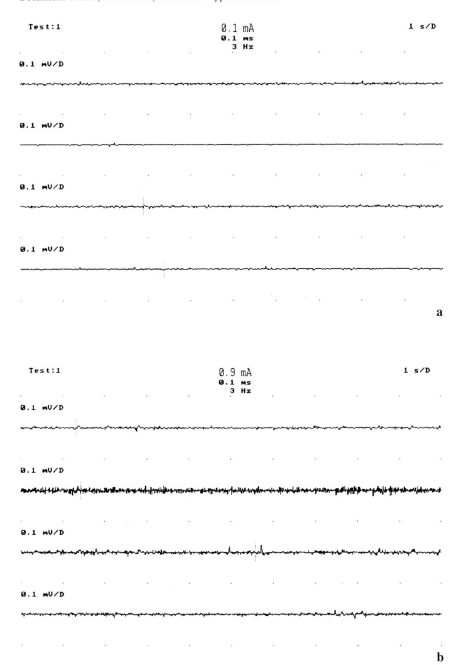

Fig. 1. (a, b) EMG surface recordings from the right and left temporal muscles (line 1 + 3), and from the right and left frontal muscles (line 2 + 4), before botulinum toxin treatment (baseline). (a) shows surface EMG of a patient with chronic TTH *without* headache during recording, (b) demonstrates EMG of a patient *with* headache during recording. Apparently, EMG surface activity is higher in the latter subject

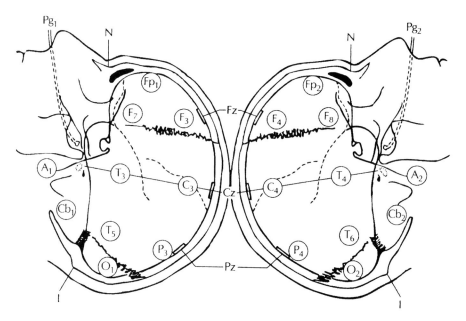

Fig. 2. International 10/20 EEG-system. Injections of DYSPORT resp. placebo have been given into the points Fp1/Fp2, F7/F8, T3/T4, T5/T6, and O1/O2. Figure modified from Ebe and Homma (1994), Fischer, Stuttgart, New York

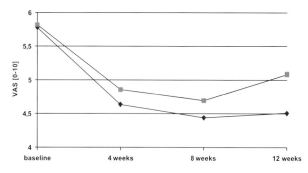

Fig. 3. Results of the Visual Analogue Scale (*VAS*) at baseline and 4, 8, and 12 weeks after treatment. No significant differences between verum and placebo treatment could be observed (modified from: [10]) ◆ Placebo; ■ Verum

References

1. Acquadro MA, Borodic GE (1994) Treatment of myofascial pain with botulinum toxin type A. Anesthesiology 80: 705–706
2. Cheshire WP, Abashian SW, Mann JD (1994) Botulinum toxin in the treatment of myofascial pain syndrome. Pain 59: 65–69
3. Göbel P, Petersen-Braun M, Soyka D (1994) The epidemiology of headache in Germany: a nationwide survey of a representative sample on the basis of the headache classification of the International Headache Society. Cephalalgia 14: 97–106
4. Haas DC (1996) Chronic post-traumatic headaches classified and compared with natural headaches. Cephalalgia 16(7): 486–493
5. Headache Classification Committee of the International Headache Society (1988) Classification and diagnostic criteria for headache disorders, cranial neuralgias and facial pain. Cephalalgia 8 [Suppl] 7: 1–96
6. Jensen R (1995) Mechanisms of spontaneous tension-type headaches: an analysis of tenderness, pain thresholds and EMG. Pain 64: 251–256
7. Langemark M, Olesen J (1987) Pericranial tenderness in tension headache. Cephalalgia 7: 249–255
8. Relja M (1997) Treatment of tension-type headache by local injection of botulinum toxin. Eur J Neurol 4 [Suppl] 2: S71–S73
9. Rollnik JD, Hierner R, Schubert M, Shen ZL, Johannes S, Tröger M, Wohlfarth K, Berger A, Dengler R (2000) Botulinum toxin treatment of cocontractions after birth-related brachial plexus lesions. Neurology 55(1): 112–114
10. Rollnik JD, Tanneberger O, Schubert M, Schneider U, Dengler R (2000) Treatment of tension-type headache with botulinum toxin type A – a double-blind placebo-controlled study. Headache 40(4): 300–305
11. Wheeler AH (1998) Botulinum toxin A, adjunctive therapy for refractory headaches associated with pericranial muscle tension. Headache 38: 468–471
12. Zwart JA, Bovim G, Sand T, Sjaastad O (1994) Tension headache: botulinum toxin paralysis of temporal muscles. Headache 34: 458–462

Part III: Extended Abstracts

Acta Neurochir (2001) [Suppl] 79: 129–143
© Springer-Verlag 2001

Abstracts Selected for Presentation at the WFNS Neuroreha-Conference Münster 2000, and on Early Rehabilitation in Maribor 2001

Does Intensive Rehabilitation Improve the Functional Outcome of Patients with Traumatic Brain Injury (TBI)? Cognitive Function Result of a Randomised Controlled Trial

X. L. Zhu, W. S. Poon, C. Chan[1], S. Wai, M. K. Tse[2], S. Chan[2], S. Yiu[2], S. Tang[2], K. Fung, C. Y. Pang, A. Chan[3], E. Lai[4], and D. Cheung[5]

[1] Neurosurgical Unit, Prince of Wales Hospital, the Chinese University of Hong Kong
[2] Department of Surgery, Prince of Wales Hospital, the Chinese University of Hong Kong
[3] Department of Occupational Therapy, Prince of Wales Hospital, the Chinese University of Hong Kong
[4] Department of Physiotherapy, Prince of Wales Hospital, the Chinese University of Hong Kong
[5] Department of Speech Therapy, Prince of Wales Hospital, the Chinese University of Hong Kong

Background and Objectives: We have carried out a randomized trial to test the efficacy of intensive rehabilitation for patients with TBI. The result showed that significantly more patients in the study group achieved full Functional Independent Measure (FIM) and good Glasgow Outcome Scale (GOS) at 3 months but the controlled group caught up in subsequent months [1]. Here we report the cognitive function outcome of the same study.

Methods: In this randomized trial with the assessors blind, two groups of patients received different intensity of rehabilitation (2 versus 4 hours per day). GOS, FIM and Neurobehavioral Cognitive Status Examination (NCSE) were assessed monthly for six months and bimonthly up to one year.

Results: 68 patients with moderate and severe TBI, aged 12–65 years, were analyzed. There was no significant difference between the two groups in scores of individual item of NCSE, total NCSE scores and FIM cognitive scores. There was a weak trend of more patients achieving full NCSE and full FIM cognitive scores in the study (intensive) group but not statistically significant.

Conclusion: This study demonstrated that intensive rehabilitation improved the early functional outcome of patients with moderate and severe TBI. However, the functional improvement (GOS) was not reflected by the cognitive function assessment by NCSE and FIM. This may be due to the low ceiling of both measures, or the combined effect of motor, cognitive and psychological factors of the patients.

Reference

1. Zhu XL, Poon WS, Chan C *et al* (1999) Does intensive rehabilitation improve the functional outcome of patients with traumatic brain injury (TBI)? One year result of a prospective randomized trial. Presented at the International Conference on Recent Advances in Neurotraumatology (ICRAN), November 20–23. Taipei, Taiwan

Post-Traumatic Vegetative States: Cost of Care

F. Danze, P. Rigaux, D. Darriet, B. Veys, A. Weber, and Ph. Lourdel
Neuro-Rehabilitation Department, Helio Marin/ Groupe Hopale Berck Sur Mer, Cedex, France

Objectives: Post-traumatic vegetative state (VS) have a reputation of causing heavy expenses on the society. This analysis is to calculate the precise cost of care in a neuro-rehabilitation department.

Methods/Patients: A data base has been created with 515 patients having been in a coma of 6 hours or more, and admitted over 12 consecutive years for rehabilitation. The data collected were: age, consciousness level on admission, Glasgow Outcome Score on leaving; amount of care, appointments and complementary exams; length of stay and daily rate in the different departments, to help calculate the average daily rate (ADR) and the total rate of hospitalization (TRH).

Results: For the 266 victims of traumatic brain injury the ADR was 1696 FF (258 Euro) and the TRH 702.000 FF (107.019 Euro) (FF 1990). By a factorial analysis of multiple correspondences (FAMC), these values varied according to age, the degree of consciousness on admission, the length of the unconsciousness period and the GOS on leaving. Among the 52 patients leaving in VS, ADR was 1237 FF (189 euro) for chronic VS and 1498 FF (228 euro) for the «non-chronic».

Discussion/Conclusion: These results cannot easily be compared to any existing literature data which remain global. On the other hand they are comparable to the data of the analytical accountancy of the Neuro-Rehabilitation Department for 1997, which estimated the daily cost of care at 1200–1250 FF (183–191 Euro) for a stabilized patient, dependent, conscious or not, and 1600–1700 FF (244–259 Euro) for a non-stabilized patient, conscious or not, dependent or not. According to an average daily cost of 1600 FF (244 Euro), an annual prevalence of 2/100.000, and a population of 57 millions French people, the annual cost of care for the VS would be 666 millions FF (102 millions Euro), that is 0,13% of the 526 billions FF spent on medical care and equipment in France (of which 1/3 could be accounted for by VS of traumatic origin that is 222 millions FF) (data 1990). The extent of the expenses on the society should be counterbalanced by the importance of the stakes for the individual. The calculated costs allow a person in chronic VS to continue to live with dignity. They allow too a person in VS to take advantage of a possible neurological and functional improvement, with the hope of the best familial, social and vocational re-integration.

Psychotherapeutic Aspects on Early Neurorehabilitation in ICU

H. Holzer

University Klinik Graz, Department of Medical Psychology and Psychotherapy, Graz, Austria

For many years the first author was a nurse at the intensive care unit (ICU) at the Department of Neurosurgery in Graz. At the same time she completed a degree in education and trained in psychotherapy, focusing on logotherapy and existential analysis. With this background she changed much in the way patients are cared for in the ICU. Her training, knowledge and psychotherapeutic approach still influence the way we do things in the unit, which the coauthor directs.

Most of the patients in the unit are unconscious or in a state of altered consciousness. Unconsciousness seems easy to define in medical terms. But ever new facets of consciousness and unconsciousness make it almost impossible to define a person in his completeness and unity. As a result, consciousness and unconsciousness mean different things to different people, based on personal experience and knowledge. We always find it a little hard to begin from the fact that a person who we classify as unconscious is a person like you or me. And if we begin from the assumption that the unconscious person has no mental capabilities, we see no sense in addressing these mental faculties. Minimal movements or expressions remain unnoticed. We deny the unconscious person any capability to feel or experience. But beginning from the hypothesis that the unconscious person is a deficient entity that feels nothing and realizes nothing and just lies there lifeless has dire consequences for the interaction.

It leads to the assumption that we cannot communicate with the unconscious patient. We deny his existence as a person and do not communicate with him. We take care of him but do not touch him. We do not think it makes sense to try. The existential analytic concept of a person, his underlying being as deducted from a philosophical theorem, appears helpful for interacting with the unconscious person. According to Frankel, a psychophysical dysfunction can lead to an inability of the spiritual person behind the psychophysical organism to express himself. But as long as I don't address the spiritual person I can't reach him therapeutically. The patient in sickness is a distortion of the true person. Care providers would not be confronted with a spiritually and physically broken apparatus, but would see the human and the spiritual being in the sick person. Only if we see the person as a holistic entity with a range of levels of consciousness and corresponding abilities to feel and to express himself, and only if we adjust to his level of communication, will we be able to interact with him.

Critical care medicine symbolizes the possible and stands for control. This leads to unrealistic and overdrawn expectations that we cannot meet. The working environment is tense, the threat of an alarm is ever present. There is pressure for success and danger of failure. The ICU is seen as an elite unit, but is often mistrusted a bit by the remainder of the hospital. The nursing staff is under psychological and physical pressure. The emotional and spiritual aspect of care is often delegated to the female nurses (*probably because we expect a maternal caring instinct of them*).

We can communicate with the unconscious patient only if we are aware of our own weaknesses, needs and fears. It makes sense to provide therapeutic support to caregivers to avoid burn out, which is common among physicians and nursing staff. The goal should be to help the staff to reach a true existential concept. This is necessary for them to take responsibility for their actions, because the challenges vary from person to person and from hour.

The existential analytical diagnosis comprises the phenomenologic picture and the binding to a theory. Taking the patient's history helps the staff get to know him. The staff knows little or nothing of the patient's personal habits, likes and dislikes, rhythms, fears, problems, familial ties or personal history. The patient is accepted as he appears, provided that the staff's own ideas and biases are excluded.

In the existential analysis, the unconscious person has deficits. This raises the question of what the patient needs to counter the deficit, so as to recover his independence. The personal interaction is at the center of existential analytical treatment. *This means that the person who is the patient becomes aware of the person who is the caregiver.* In this concept there are no routine care measures, there are only individual therapeutic actions. The guiding principle is to adapt routines to patients, not patients to routines. We try to look not only at the patient's physical status and level of consciousness but also at his remaining motor or sensory capabilities.

Early neurorehabilitation for patients with head injuries should start at the scene of the accident. This usually doesn't happen, and it doesn't happen often in the receiving intensive care unit (ICU) either. There are a lot of arguments against early neurorehabilitation, for example the fear increasing the intracranial pressure in the early and sensitive phase of the injury. But this is not the case and contrary to modern concepts of neurorehabilitation in the acute phase. Another problem is that patients with severe brain injuries are still taken to and accepted by hospitals with no infrastructure for early neurorehabilitation. At the Department of Neurosurgery of the University of Graz, we try to follow the principles of early neurorehabilitation.

In Austria there is a nation-wide plan for early neurorehabilitation. But depending on the regional hospital organization the implementation of this plan is in its infancy. There is a requirement of 25–35 early rehabilitation beds (rehabilitation category B beds) for brain injuries per million population per year.

There is a wide gap between the ideals of rehabilitation concepts and reality. Also, in Austria accidents are taken care of by different insurance plans depending on the setting in which they occur. Patients with job injuries receive intense rehabilitation all the way until they can resume employment. All costs are covered. In contrast, injuries not related to employment, including the traffic accidents unrelated to work are covered during the initial care. However, transfer to appropriate rehabilitation centres is often extremely delayed. Self-help groups and political activities have improved things, but the high costs of rehabilitation render many plans unimplemented.

I do not mean to sound negative. But I do want to critically evaluate the status quo and emphasize the importance of early and longer term neurorehabilitation. Regional peculiarities in Austria lead to white areas on maps of neurorehabilitation coverage in our country. This is true for brain injuries as well as for other conditions of the central nervous system with neurological deficits.

Neuropsychological View on Early Neurorehabilitation – View from Denmark

A.-L. Christensen

Neuropsychology, University of Copenhagen, Denmark

The Needs of the Neurotraumatic Patient: For the patient who has suffered an acute neurotrauma, the immediate need is clearly an active and thorough medical care, where all means available to the neurosurgeon and the staff in the intensive care unit have to be considered.

The immediate target for treatment is thus the brain as the controlling organ of the organism. However, is this patient treated as an object and not as soon as possible understood as an individual person, it cannot be claimed that the best possible early rehabilitation has been provided.

Treatment of the brain as the controlling organ of the mind has to be included.

The Team Treating the Neurotraumatic Patient: The members of the multi- or interdisciplinary team have to be experts in medical care, in neurosurgery and neurology, in nursing and in occupational- and physiotherapy collaborating in the initial treatment of the neurotrauma patient, assisted as soon as possible by experts educated within the fields of brain functioning, i.e. experts in psychology/ neuropsychology, in education and in speech- and language therapy.

In the multi- or interdisciplinary team it is the specific knowledge and skills of each member that define his/her contribution to the treatment of the patient and the role played in relation to and in agreement with the other team members. Included in the definition is also the demand to collaborate with all others to ensure shared information and common strategies within the various approaches.

The Role of the Neuropsychologist: In relation to the *patient* an important task for the neuropsychologist in the very early stage is participation in the evaluation of the level of consciousness, often in combination with considerations regarding kind and amount of stimulation.

The goal to be able to establish contact to the patient and to provide information and reassurance can be promoted by repeated and daily visits to the patient's bedside.

The establishment of a relationship to the patient's *relatives* is a natural part of the same kind of efforts. The demands and needs of the relatives have to be met with a psychological understanding of the situation they are experiencing at the same time as it is reassuring for them to provide the information that is needed for the most appropriate treatment of the patient.

Integrating all collected information about the patient from the various sources available, that can be added to the general information in the patient's records, is another task, important for the whole treatment process.

Also contact to nurses and other members of the team regarding psychological characteristics of the patient's function and of his/her reactions can be a valuable part of the neuropsychologist's work in the early phase.

A task that the neuropsychologist traditionally is asked to perform as early as possible is a neuropsychological assessment.

The daily visits to the patient's bedside can be of help in deciding the right time for this investigation at the same time as they provide the possibility to inform the patient about what is going to take place. It should be the goal of the neuropsychologist to create a relationship of thrust to ensure motivation and collaboration, so if it is needed this information has to be repeated.

The initial phase of an assessment should be oriented towards obtaining information about the patient's own feelings, his/her past experiences and also his/her feelings about the current situation with the purpose of providing insight in the level of consciousness, in the patient's complaints, in his/her memory function and over-all personality.

Several tools exist for assessment. It is recommended to carefully plan what tests to use in the individual case. Usually a hypothesis can be made on the background of neurological findings, which makes it possible to illuminate preserved as well as disturbed functions within a time span, that can ensure that the disturbances are primary, not secondary caused by tiredness.

The Luria Neuropsychological Investigation (LNI) contains tests that can be performed at the patient's bedside, and is an investigation that has proven to be a useful tool in the hands of experienced neuropsychologists in the acute stage of brain injury. It is structured on the basis of knowledge about brain function, and the terminology is neurological, providing a common language for the interdisciplinary team. Brain function is examined in simple as well as complex tasks and the results can be summarized in syndromes, comparable to objective neurological and neuroradiological findings.

The report describing the neuropsychological functioning should contain information important for the planning and initiation of rehabilitation as well as some prognostic considerations. It should be discussed by the team, and findings and observations from other disciplines incorporated with the aim of planning a collaborative intervention, sharing tasks according to expertise and experience.

Early Rehabilitative Treatment: Attempts at remediating function should be initiated as early as possible in combination with providing continuous support and information.

A. R. Luria recommended *deinhibition* in the acute stage, by which he meant demanding a sudden reaction of the patient, that could not be performed voluntarily. *Stressing intact functions* have proven useful and so have *providing feed back* and *changing conditions during task solutions in an interactive way. Repetition of tasks* is meaningful, especially if improvements are integrated in a dynamic development of the progress taking place.

The principles are uniform and can be applied in the various therapeutic connections.

Collaboration of the Interdisciplinary Team: In order to ensure the optimal effect of the treatment provided by the team members there need to be a continuous representation of at least one member of each discipline in conferences, referring and discussing up-to-date information and integrating this in the further rehabilitative planning.

Also discharge performance and transfer of the patient to proper continued treatment are tasks involving the interdisciplinary team. At transfer a comprehensive report containing integrated plans based on diagnosis and treatment results should follow the patient.

Summarizing: The role of the neuropsychologist in the interdisciplinary team during early rehabilitation is multifacetted, although constantly concerned with issues related to the psychological functioning of the injured brain and the patient's reactions to the consequences of the injury. In relationship to the *patient* the main tasks are to provide continuous support and understanding, to evaluate intact as well as disturbed functions, cognitively, emotionally and socially.

Participation in the planning of the optimal rehabilitative course provided by each of the team members and by the combined group is mandatory.

Availability for the patient's *relatives* should be a part of the role but also *availability* to be a partner in discussions with the aim of *assisting all other team members* in the parts of their clinical work that is related to *psychological theory and insight* must be included in the work of the neuropsychologist.

Neurorehabilitation – the Danish Concept

A. Nordenbo

Hvidovre University Hospital, Denmark

Background: In 1997 The Danish National Board of Health recommended to intensify the treatment of the severely brain injured. Subsequently it was decided to establish two departments, one in the

Western part of Denmark at Hammel Hospital of Neurorehabilitation and one in Eastern Denmark at Hvidovre University Hospital. The units should provide early, intensive multidisciplinary treatment of the severely brain injured.

Denmark with its 5.2 million inhabitants was estimated to have 600 severely injured patients per year and of these approximately 100 needed treatment in a specialized unit.

In October 2001 the unit at Hvidovre Hospital was opened and now it comprises 20 beds, 14 for adults from 16 years and up and 6 for children from 2–15 years. All members of the staff went on a one month teaching course before opening. During the course teaching of the medical aspects was provided as well as courses and practical exercises in creating and working in teams. A four day introductory course in the principles of Affolter, Bobath and Coombes (ABC – concept) was included. The rehabilitation principles of the unit are founded on this concept.

Admission: The patients are admitted directly from the neurosurgical intensive care unit as soon as they are on spontaneous ventilation and no longer need neurosurgical treatment and observation. It is important that the patients can be received without unnecessary delay. At the moment only patients with a traumatic etiology are admitted.

Many patients are multitraumatized and skills of semi-intensive care as well as skills needed for long-term neurological rehabilitations have to be demanded from the team. The advantage of admitting the patients for rehabilitation at such an early stage is however that treatment starting early and intensively is the best way to avoid complications such as malnutrition and contractures and the best way to restore cognitive functions.

Teams: Before admission a primary team consisting of two from the nursing staff, one physiotherapist and one occupational therapist are appointed. Among those a team-coordinator is chosen. This primary team has the responsibility for the day to day planning of the rehabilitation and the coordinator has an additional responsibility for coordination with the larger team and for more long-term planning. The larger team includes a neurologist, a neuropsychologist, a speech therapist, a social worker and for the older children, a school teacher. The team-work is interdisciplinary which includes that common goals are made after discussion, that borders between disciplines are softened and that the members also meet informally during the day. Coordination of the rehabilitation *as a whole* is intended.

Family Support: The primary team and the doctor meet with the family on the first day of admission for the first team-meeting. Consultations with the neuropsychologist and social worker are organized routinely. A family support group which meet once a month has just started and the results so far are promising. Team-meetings with the larger team are arranged every 4–6 weeks.

Rating Scales: A battery of ratings scales are applied including Glasgow coma scale, EFA (early functional ability test), FIM score (functional independence measure) and Rancho Los Amigos global test of cognition. A database is under development in corporation with Hammel Hospital of Neurorehabilitation. These ratings form a base for future research at the unit.

Experiences: The organisation and start of the unit has been carefully planned and the one month introductory course for all disciplines has made a foundation of invaluable importance. Getting started was not easy and interdisciplinary team work is not being built in one week, one month but hopefully as it seems in one year! There is a current need for follow-up and further education and financial resources have been calculated in the budget for the next few years.

Although interdisciplinary team work may sometimes seem difficult and time consuming, the benefit for the patient, the family, the rehabilitation process and thus for the outcome, far overshadows the difficulties that appear. Interdisciplinary team work is thus strongly recommended.

Early Neurorehabilitation – Neurosurgical View
M. Lipovšek
Neurosurgical Department, General Hospital Maribor, Maribor, Slovenia

Objectives: In the primary stages of administering to a brain damaged patient or treating a patient after acute brain disorder, it is the Neurosurgeon, but also the Neurologist and the Intensive Care Physician, who are principally involved, applying medical criteria first and foremost. They will, however, be keeping in mind from the outset, that early Neurorehabilitation also requires the *early* participation of different experts, if optimum results for the well-being of the patient are ultimately to be achieved.

Material and Methods: The main responsibility for harmonious team-work and the management of the team, must remain with the physician, who is obliged to link up and co-ordinate the work of these experts of different professional backgrounds. The team in Maribor consists of the Neurosurgeon, the nursing staff, a physiotherapist and clinical speech pathologist. A Neuropsychologist is not available in the hospital.

Prigatano has pointed out that for a holistic approach, which involves early Neurorehabilitation, adequate surroundings must be first created. This does not mean solely the provision of sufficient time or suitable space, but also refers to creating a whole climate of credibility and trust, in which all those who attended the patient are convinced and genuinely believe that such a treatment is necessary and beneficial. This is not always easy. Matters can be complicated in so many different ways:

- The patient, as the result of brain damage, may be in a state of unconsciousness.
- Consciousness may be impaired to a greater or lesser degree.
- The patient may not be able to communicate at all.
- The patient's breathing may be dependant on a respirator in the ICU and while attached to all the monitoring devices, the priority will be to carry out the procedures required just to prevent deterioration.

The medical staff would be called upon to deal with all such complex situations. However, the patient's consciousness may be not so adversely altered as to prevent us from recognising some measure of meaningful motor reaction or correct motor response to touching, speech or other sensory stimulation of the patient. When such response appears logical (particularly if it can be repeated), it can not be attributed merely to reflex reaction, as it so often is, but should be classified as the patient's *optimal functional ability*. It is actually astonishing how we can detect, in patient with altered consciousness, signs of communicative ability, given patience and a fine-tuned attentiveness on our part. It is usually noticed in the course of careful nursing care: while performing suction of the respiratory tract, the inserting of a gastric tube or just turning the patient over in bed etc. We have to ask ourselves how great, in fact, is the patient's capacity for sustaining thought process, experiencing and understanding, despite a brain lesion which may be requiring artificial ventilation or other pharmacological interventions, all of which may render the patient immobile. We certainly make a big error if we discuss the

Table 1. *Early Neurorehabilitation – The Average Yearly Number of Treated Patients in the Period from 1996 till 2000*

1995–2000	Department	Sex		Total
		Female	Male	
	Neurology	67	77	144
	Neurosurgery	22	26	48
	Total	89	103	192

situation in front of the patient believing him/her to be incapable of comprehension. Clearly, the early stage requires, above all, medical management, especially where there is severe brain injury. However it is nevertheless prudent to obtain the information about his/her capability of awareness and communication as early as possible. The assessment can be non-verbal and should be carried out by a Neuropsychologist or, as in our case, by a speech pathologist who is well versed in other cognitive and neurological disorders. Careful primary management and successful medical treatment can lead to early functional assessment of the remaining activities, which will then serve us well in the subsequent Neurorehabilitation programme. The physician's duty is, therefore, to balance constantly the procedures which are tailored individually and which should prevent any secondary complications. In this he is greatly helped by regular reports from the members of the team.

Results: The average number of patients treated in the last five years is presented in Table 1

The physician's duty is to balance the procedures in the early stage of hospital management which must be tailored individually and which should prevent any secondary complications. In this enterprise for Neurorehabilitation, the Neurosurgeon's particular concerns are:

Taking into account up-to date guidelines on the subject. These will help to direct medical management towards gradually establishing the physiological environment in the brain. Results obtained from monitoring, computers, laboratory and roentgen analyses should not occupy us to such an extent that we are found «to be 'treating' the screen, films and laboratory findings». Regular physical examination brings us into close contact with the patient and helps to evaluate the presence of functional optimal ability. Improvement depends on the state of consciousness and other preserved functions, but the manner of treatment, which may take time, is also a matter of consequence. The time factor is important. The right choice of particular procedures in an appropriate given time span, is what determines the quality of our work.

The state of the Respiratory and Cardiovascular Systems. WE have to endeavour to prevent infection but if, despite all efforts, we fail then, for example, a balanced decision has to be made regarding tracheostomy, which can delay and prolong the teamwork for weeks and months.

The feeding, gastroduodenal tube, i.v. fluids, micturition etc. Tube feeding, an unnatural procedure in itself, may be concealing, for example, some impediment on the local level in the oral cavity or the problem may be central. Owing to impaired consciousness, damage to the brain stem, apraxia, or there may just be a more complex cognitive disorder responsible. From the Neurorehabilitation point of view the oral cavity is an important, if it can be described, 'crossroads', where three vital activities meet: breathing, swallowing and speech.

Nursing procedures which are the domain of the nursing staff. Apart from regular medical obligations, it must be emphasised the importance of nursing care, prevention of thrombosis, bedsores etc., which all contribute to a faster general activation and hopefully, eventual verticalisation of the patient. These factors all play a significant part in moving forward the concurrent work of the Neurophysiotherapist and Clinical speech pathologist who, in absence of a Neuropsychologist in Maribor, is not only responsible for re-establishing verbal communication but, if this fails, achieving at least a modicum of meaningful communication, which would facilitate the patient's return home and back into society.

The patient's relatives. They are in a distressed state and invariably anxious for information. This can be given by any member of the team, but only from the aspect of his/her own individual field of expertise. It is the Neurosurgeon or Neurologist who is in possession of all the facts and has therefore an overall view, who is responsible for maintaining and providing all information about the patient's progress.

Discussion: Despite optimal plans and programmes we have to keep in mind that Early Neurorehabilitation can not *guarantee* the return to a «normal pre-injury state». The majority of medical personnel regard the term 'rehabilitation' to mean the process and events which take place following medical treatment and, as a rule, in another institution. Not infrequently such programmes start many weeks and months after acute brain disorder has occurred. Our experience with Early Neurorehabilitation suggests that we achieve a much better overall outcome than do rehabilitation programmes which commence later, after a period of time has elapsed. If we have conducted Early Neurorehabilitation, it is much easier to transfer the patients to the one and only Institute of Rehabilitation we have, for further treatment. The Slovenian central rehabilitation Institute does not accept patients who have no ability to communicate, have severe cognitive impairment and/or the complex neurological disorder which prevents a patient from attaining a sitting position. These patients end up in various nursing homes. Early Neurorehabilitation sadly fails those who have been diagnosed as being in a vegetative state, but it has to be stressed that even questions of this nature have nowadays become far more polemical than previously.

Favourable and successful team work obviously requires broader analyses. WE would like to invite teams from other hospitals, with similar ambitions and possibilities, to study the importance and the need for Early Neurorehabilitation. Analyses of a greater number of patients treated in this manner, might help and clarify many of the questions which are frequently raised.

Conclusion: A patient with acute brain disorder should have multidisciplinary treatment of which Early Neurorehabilitation plays a significant role. In the course of such quality management it is possible to observe clinical and functional changes with more clarity. Multidisciplinary approach gains deeper insight and understanding of the recovery from (even) severe functional impairment to the state where regular rehabilitation programme can continue after the discharge from the ICU or Neurosurgical/Neurological department. Team work is necessary in every medical department which takes up acute traumatic brain injury and neurological emergencies. Therefore it is recommended that Early Neurorehabilitation should become an indispensable part of medical management following acute or post-traumatic brain damage.

References

1. Stajnko M, Lipovšek M (1999) Early Neurorehabilitation. In: KRH von Wild, V Hömberg, Annegret Ritz (Hrsg) Das schädelhirnverletzte Kind. Motorische Rehabilitation – Qualitätsmanagement (1999) W. Zuckscherdt Verlag, München Bern Wien New York

The Torneo Project for Professional Reintegration of People with Acquired Brain Injury

Dr. Engelien Lannoo and Wilfried Brusselmans

Center for Locomotor and Neurological Rehabilitation, University Hospital, De Pintelaan, Gent Belgium

Introduction: Although brain injuries often result in permanent unemployment, many survivors remain motivated to work and identify it as a primary rehabilitation goal. The European Torneo project offered the opportunity to realise a specialised training program for professional rehabilitation of brain injured people who are functionally independent in activities of daily living and want to return to work or school.

Methods: The transnational cooperation allowed the development of uniform methods for vocational and prevocational rehabilitation of brain injured people. One of the main goals of the project was the evaluation and training of vocational abilities in real work environments. In order to realise this, job trials were introduced. These could take place in one of the departments of the University Hospital, such as the gardeners, the kitchen, the administration department, the child care, etc.; or on the work floor of an external employer. The job trials were introduced progressively, starting with a few half days a week.

Results: During the project, a total of 46 brain injured individuals entered the program. The majority were males, with a lower education, who suffered from traumatic brain injury. Mean age was 32 years, mean coma duration was 14 days. The time interval between injury and program entry varied from a few months to approximately 5 years, with a mean time interval of nine months. The mean duration of the treatment program was 3 months.

Of the 36 patients who had finished the program by the end of the project in October 1997, more than half had achieved a positive result: 11 were able to return to work, 2 patients worked as volunteers, 6 patients could return to school, and 1 patient was following a vocational education program. Three patients who had not yet finished the program yet were doing a job trial with a potential employer and had good chances of future employment there.

When the 20 patients achieving a positive result were compared with the 16 who did not, we found significant differences between both groups on the time interval between injury and program entry, in favour of those patients starting the program earlier. We also found a difference regarding level of education. Patients with a higher education achieved better results than those with lower education. With regard to age, gender, coma length and duration of treatment, no differences were found.

Conclusion: Through the participation in the European Torneo project, a specialized vocational rehabilitation program was developed for people with acquired brain injuries to ameliorate their chances on a succesful professional reintegration. By starting this professional rehabilitation as soon as possible following injury, the duration of work incapacity was kept to a minimum. Moreover, the results of the project indicated that the chances on a succesful professional reintegration diminish as the period of work incapacity is getting longer. Therefore it is important to start professional rehabilitation as soon as possible following functional rehabilitation.

References

1. Crepeau F, Scherzer P (1993) Predictors and indicators of work status after traumatic brain injury: a meta-analysis. Neuropsychol Rehab 3: 5–35
2. Dikmen S, Temkin N, Machamer J *et al* (1994) Employment following traumatic head injuries. Arch Neurol 51: 177–186
3. Ponsford J, Olver J, Curran C *et al* (1995) Prediction of employment status 2 years after traumatic brain injury. Brain Inj 9: 11–20

B.N.I., a New Tool for Rapid Evaluation of Higher Cerebral Functions of Traumatic Brain Injured Patients

M. Marinescu, R. Rusina, Z. S. de Boisgeheneuc, and J. L. Truelle

Service de Neurologie, Hôpital Foch, Suresnes Cedex, France

Objectives: The rapid and global evaluation of higher cerebral functions has a major interest in the approach of traumatic brain injured patients. Until now, it didn't exist, excluding the Mini Mental Status (M.M.S.), a test which allies rapidity, sensibility and pertinence. The B.N.I. (Barrow Neurological Institute) test, validated and published by Prigatano [1, 2] in 1995, appears to be a test which could modify this.

Patients and Method: We used the B.N.I. test in its French version [3] for evaluating the cognitive performances of 70 traumatic brain injured patients. Their results were compared to those of 100 non-traumatic brain injured, of 100 normal subjects and of 100 patients which had psychiatric attempt. A viability study was made.

Results: The results show the greater sensibility of the B.N.I. test (85%), compared to the M.M.S. results for the same groups, particularly for the mild traumatic brain injuries where the sensibility was 95%. It has the object of evaluating the emotional status and the self-awareness of troubles, at the same time as the cognitive functions evaluated by this type of test (language, orientation, memory, visiospatial functions …) The mean time needed for passing the test was 11,8 minutes.

Conclusion: 25 years after the M.M.S., the B.N.I. test is a real progress in the global and rapid evaluation of higher cerebral functions in a medical consultation, particularly for traumatic and non traumatic brain injured patients.

References

1. Prigatano G (1991) BNI screen for higher cerebral functions. BNI Qu 7: 2–9
2. Prigatano G, Amin K (1993) Validity studies for the BNI screen for higher cerebral functions, BNI Qu 9: 2–9
3. Truelle JL, Joseph PA, Mazaux JM, Manning L, Prigatano G. Une version française du B.N.I., test d'évaluation rapide des fonctions supérieures (under press)

Thoughts on Early Neuro Rehabilitation (ENR) in Germany and Own Experience

E. Ortega-Suhrkamp and S. Mundiyanapurath

Asklepios Schloßberg-Klinik, Bad König, Germany

Summary: Since 1993 an average of 400 patients annually have been treated in our clinic after most severe acquired brain damage (traumatic brain injury, intracerebral haemorrhage, subarachnoid haemorrhage, hypoxia and severe stroke) strictly following the guidelines as published by the German Task Force in 1993 (quality of structure, procedure and outcome). Treatment is effected in an interdisciplinary team with the staffing situation as indicated in the guidelines. The outcome is measured by means of scales such as

Table 1. *Classification of the Phases A–F (Chain of Rehabilitation)*

Phase A: Acute care
Phase B: Early intensive
          Unawareness, fully dependent
Phase C: Partial Unawareness
          Partially cooperative
Phase D: Mobilized, cooperative
Phase E: Professional Training for Re-employment
Phase F: Nursing care

Table 2. *Criteriae for Finishing Early Rehabilitation*

A: If the following criteriae for transfer into further rehabilitation
      are reached:
Vegetative stability
Partial mobilization (i.e. wheel chair)
Ways for communication and interaction
Improved cognitive function
Following simple orders, taking an active part in simple activities
      and enduring 30 minutes of exercise within one therapeutic unit
      several times a day, with rest periods as needed
Decreasing behavior problems
Ability to function within a small group, showing culturally
      accepted social behavior, and
The amount of nursing care must be less than 4 hours per day
B: If, over the course of several months of undisturbed therapy,
      there is no essential improvement, and if medical judgment
      excludes any improvement in the near future.

Table 3. *Staffing Situation for a 20-Bed-Unit*

Nurses 1 : 0,4–0,75
Speech Therapist 1 : 7,5
Physio- and Occupational-Therapist 1 : 4
Therapeutic Pedagogue 1 : 7,5
Social Worker 1 : 15
Psychologist 1 : 15
Medical Doctors: 1 Consultant of Neurology, Neurosurgery or
      Neuropediatrics, 1 Assistent Consultant and 2 Attending
      Physicians
1 Medical Technician
1 Secretary and 1,5 Ward Aids

Coma Remission Scale, Functional Independence Measure, Disability Rating Scale and GOS.

Objectives: In 1993, the Task Force "Early Neurological-Neurosurgial Rehabilitation" published "Recommendations for ENR", which included aspects of structure-, procedure- and outcome-based quality (1, Tab. 1 Phase B and C). These recommendations were accepted by insurance companies, politicians and rightful claimants and were then translated into the structuring of professional Early Rehabilitation Departments at responsible clinics throughout the country. The great advantage which resulted is that now, all over Germany, we offer a variety of Early Rehabilitation Centers, which all work according to the same concept with only minor differences, and thus, are comparable in terms of quality management.

Material and Methods: We were among one of the very first neurological rehabilitation departments in Germany, starting as early as 1989. So, we were privileged to contribute our own experiences and ideas to this concept.

Early Rehabilitation is an independent, therapeutic concept of diagnostic, rehabilitative and psychosocial measures. Among all therapeutic procedures involved, ENR holds a special place because of the severe peripheral and complex cerebral damage of the nervous system with secondary disorders of all organic systems – may it be caused by brain injury, haemorrhage, stroke, brain tumor, hypoxia or other acute brain disorders, Guillain-Barré-Syndrome and so on.

Early Rehabillitation is right at the beginning of the so called "Chain of Rehabilitation" (table 1) and has its place between intensive care and further medical rehabilitation. Therefore, the essential aspects of acute care and intensive care therapy are combined with specific rehabilitative therapy. In ICU, the stabilization of vital functions has top priority. However, the primary goal of Early Rehabilitation is to begin the re-learning process of daily living competence for the patient.

The beginning of Early Rehabilitation is calculated individually. It depends on the severity and clinical progress of the brain damage as well as on the general state of the patient. As soon as life-threatening complications have ceased, vegetative functions are stabilized and the danger of acute ICP is excluded, then Early Rehabilitation should be started, alongside acute care therapy, even while the patient is still in the Intensive Care Unit. The patient should be transferred into the Early Rehabilitation Department as soon as possible. Partial dependency of ventilation, neurological intensive care monitoring, central venous catheter, parenteral nutrition and blocked tracheotomy tube are not excluding criteria for transfer into any Early Rehabilitation Department.

The targets of Early Rehabilitation are supporting and enhancing the course of spontaneous remission, encouraging all existing potential rehabilitation to its optimum, considering the plasticity of the brain, early identifying and removing of complications such as hydrocephalus, contractures, pressure sores and osteoporosis, for example, and taking countermeasures toward behavior problems.

While in therapy the neurological and neuropsychological improvement is observed clinically and measured by an assessment by scales. In team sessions it is decided if the patient may pass on directly after an intervall therapy into further rehabilitation or into home care.

Early Rehabilitation is stopped according to up-to-date standards of medical experience as showed in table 2.

Early Rehabilitation can take anytime from a few weeks up to six months and more. Due to short financial resources, some federal states are suggesting an average rehabilitation period of only 60 days. There are special criteria for admission, discharge and duration of therapy. Contrary to adults not only the recovery of pre-existing abilities and skills is to re-learn but even more so the recovery of their pre-traumatic stage of development.

Even room and technical capacity are prescribed in our concept. Briefly the wards must provide enough room capacity in order to store and use all monitoring devices safely, as well as moving the patient into a wheelchair with sufficient space for mobility.

It goes without saying that due to the severity of their illness, all patients need to have the option to be monitored for 24 hours covering all their vital functions: oxygen supply, emergency ventilation, ECG, blood pressure, EEG. Long-term ECG and EEG, long-term blood pressure monitoring, emergency laboratory, neurophysiological examinations, radiology, laryngoscopy, bronchoscopy, gastroscopy, sonography and Doppler sonograghy need to be readily available.

Structure of the staff: Early Rehabilitation must be well staffed and, consequently, is very expensive. A typical staffing situation for a 20-bed-unit shows *table 3*. There might be a variety of therapists, i.e. music therapists, painting therapists, nursing therapists. The Chief of Neurology bears total responsibility. She or he integrates and coordinates all rehabilitation processes, and ensures that safe quality measures are followed. The entire therapeutic team needs determined, knowledgeable and reliable leadership.

Results: Working in an interdisciplinary team optimizes the combined care in order to enhance each patient's abilities. This requires highly qualified staff, which by professional education, experience and psychophysical resistance, needs to be up to the task. The staff has to undergo continuous post-graduate education, specifically as well as interdisciplinary. On a regular basis, an external management consultant and psychologist comes for training on topics like how to lead conversations and discussions, how to resolve conflict, dealing with next of kin, and many other topics according to the actual need of all staff involved.

Also, an external psychologist supervises patient-orientated discussions. In my opinion, it is vital to continuously motivate, train and support all staff at all levels. Only in relaxed surroundings is the team able to treat the completely dependent patient with dignity, and to always ask themselves during therapeutic activities: "How would I feel if I were the patient?" If these requirements are met – then, and only then! – the patient is truly the central focus of the team and this is the key objective of the concept. A first-rate concept by itself will never have a successful result. But if this concept is carried out by a multi-disciplinary team committed to the outcome, then the concept has the greatest chance for success. The area surrounding the patient consists of family, nursing staff, therapeutic staff, and of doctors. As a rule, in the beginning of ENR the patient needs close monitoring of all vital parameters. At this stage, the immediate objectives are defined in the first team discussion according to investigations of sensomotoric and cognitive functions, and of relative strength. Every patient has **a** treatment plan with clearly defined goals. Frequently found immediate objectives at the beginning of Early Rehabilitation might be spontaneous respiration, encouragement of vigilance, stabilizing of circulation, creating an atmosphere free of anxiety, along with facial-oral stimulation to develop swallowing and speaking. The caring team members at this early stage consist of nursing staff, physiological and occupational therapists as well as doctors. The assigned and documented objectives are checked and corrected. More precisely, the assignments are adapted rather than merely corrected, when the set goal is reached. For example initiating an early dialogue by means of music; promoting perception through training on a treadmill; developing spontaneous activity; reducing perception disturbance; painting; re-learning personal hygiene with hand-on-hand instruction, early cognitive promotion as well as working in small groups for social re-integration – just to name a few possibilities of adapted goals. We start very early with the training of daily-living activities such as taking breakfast or lunch together with other patients as well as playing in small activity groups for social re-integration and reduction of behavior problems. At our clinic, these are a combined effort of general nursing staff and nursing pedagogues, with their professional training somewhere between occupational therapists and nurses.

Discussion: The heart of the concept is teamwork with very small authority difference in hierarchy. Within our basic continuing education we include dealing with perceptionally disturbed patients, the treatment of swallowing and eating disturbances, basal stimulation, and the concept of Bobath and Kinesthetic.

Let me stress once again the importance to work with clearly defined objectives on an interdisciplinary basis at each single stage of therapy. For example about tow thirds of our patients suffer from swallowing problems. On their day of admission specially trained

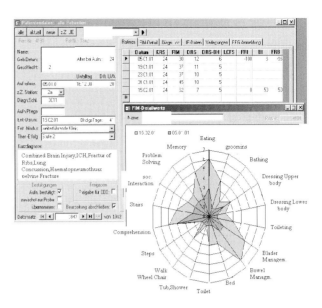

Fig. 1. Database containing the basic information of the patient, diagnosis and rating scales. FIM-scale: shows the score at the beginning of Early Rehabilitation, demonstrates the score at demission

occupational therapists check the patient and complete the "bedside-status" form, which gives the basis for the therapy needed. The therapists may even recommend a laryngoscopy.

After this initial treatment and as soon as the patient is able to swallow on stimulation, then the physio-, speech-, and nursing therapists may also start their training with the patient for swallowing and eating functions.

After 4 to 6 weeks of therapy, the long-term objectives need to be defined in a team session to determine whether the patient will be able to reach the point of moving on into further rehabilitation or whether he will remain to be dependent on nursing care.

Documentation of any stage is of utmost importance. In addition to documenting each single therapy session, we keep records on progress and therapy, as well as scales for prognosis: The Coma-Remission-Scale, which was developed by the study group on Early Rehabilitation, then the Functional Indepence Measure (FIM), Barthel Index, and the Disability Rating Scale (DRS). The updating of each patient's scales is done during our interdisciplinary team sessions. The gradings are computerized in a database containing the basic information for the patient and are available to all team members for the assessment of progress (fig. 1). The gradings also give the fundamental dates for research statistic analysis and also for annual statistics. Fig. 2 shows for example the outcome of brain injury for the year 2000.

As a general rule, the concept of Early Rehabilitation includes taking care of the patient's family as well. Particularly at the earlier stage the family feels extremely uncertain about the outcome of this illness, which one day gives rise to new hope, only to fall back into disappointment and anxiety the next day, depending on the patient's reactions. Regular talks with the doctor are necessary to help the caring family understand the illness and the various stages of it. Also, psychologists offer crisis intervention talks. Introducing the caring family to nursing and certain therapies can often be useful as it has the potential of reducing the feeling of helplessness for the family members. Full day seminars with hand-on training as well as a get-together take place. Further we offer the scope of a Wellness program. Representatives of the Protestant and Catholic Church, as in-

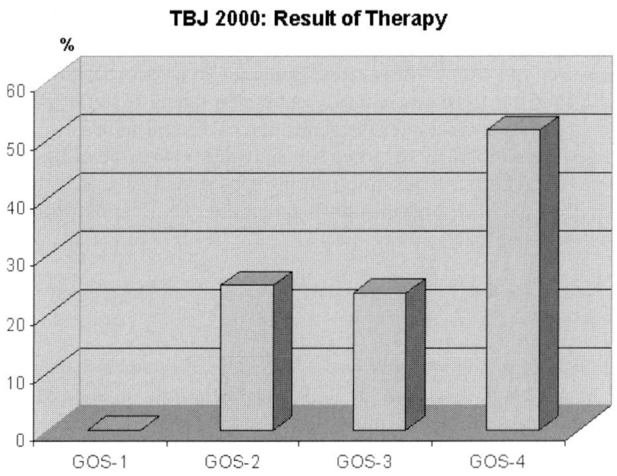

TBJ 2000: Result of Therapy

Fig. 2. Outcome of 132 patients after traumatic brain injury at the end of Early Rehabilitation: GOS 1: 0%, GOS 2: 25%, GOS 3: 23,3%, GOS 4: 51,5%, GOS 5: 0%

stitutions outside the clinic, have proved to be especially helpful in supporting the patient's family. If so desired, hotel rooms belonging to the clinic are available for the families.

Conclusion: And now to sum up, let me mention that in Germany, ER departments can be run under national health hospitals as well as in privately run rehabilitation centers. This carries one disadvantage for our concept because the medical care for severely brain damaged patients could collapse if the insurances no longer cover the cost – which might happen with the introduction of DRGs. The department of ER has to be independent with its own rooms, its own team and department head. There must be closely available specialists for other areas of support as needed, such as availability Neurosurgeons, Orthopedic or General surgeons, ENT or eye doctors, and so on.

Last not least according to the concept of ER scientific investigations must be made. These investigations consist of a close connection between fundamental science as well as practical sciences, i.e.

Clinical experimentation of medications used for brain protection
Critical examination of comastimulation therapy
Longterm studies, like single case studies and epidemological, for elaborating the prognosis and the outcome of brain damage patients.

Working according to this conception is successful. I think we have to be grateful to have had the possibility of developing a common concept of ER in Germany and we still have finances to apply for. Because of that we have the possibility to treat and support the severe brain-damaged patients on their long and painful way of re-learning life with dignity.

Reference

1. Voss A (1993) Standards der neurologisch-neurochirurgischen Frührehabilitation Ein Konzept der Arbeitsgemeinschaft Neurologische-Neurochirurgische Frührehabilitation in Fortschritte in der Neurotraumatologie und klinischen Neuropsychologie 1, Spektrum der Neurorehabilitation, Herausgeber K, von Wild HH, W Zuckschwerdt Verlag Münschen – Bern – Wien – New York, 112–120

Combating Brain Attack: Therapeutic Strategies for Patients with Subarachnoid or Intracerebral Haemorrhage of Grave Prognosis

Y. Kato, H. Sano, S. Nagahisa, S. Iwata, and T. Kanno

Department of Neurosurgery, Fujita Health University, Toyoake, Aichi, Japan

Aim: To discuss the advances in treatment strategies for the management of grade IV and V aneurysmal subarachnoid hemorrhage (SAH) and hypertensive intracerebral hematoma (HICH) and to identify the factors influencing prognosis.

Patients and Methods: The study includes 83 patients with SAH and in a poor grade (30 in grade IV and 53 in grade V) and 153 patients with HICH. Thirty-four patients in grade V SAH could only be administered CPA. The rest of the patients with SAH underwent surgical clipping (including ventricular drainage, evacuation of cerebral hematoma by jet irrigation, local dispersion of urokinase, reduced temporary occlusion time to less than 5 minutes and preservation of pial vessels) or therapeutic coil embolization. In patients demonstrating vasospasm, local intraarterial injection of papavarine was administered. Infectious complications were prevented by maintaining hypothermia. One patient with grade V SAH also underwent cerebral refrigeration for cerebral edema.

153 patients with HICH underwent hyperbaric oxygen (HBO) therapy followed by hematoma evacuation using neuroendoscope under real time CT fluoroscopy.

We have developed the real-time CT fluoroscopy which has made it possible to track target shifts during surgical procedures [1, 2]. With this instrumentation we feel that we can really achieve the ultimate aims of minimally invasive surgery ie precise target localization and surgical procedure with no injury to surrounding brain tissue. When data for 360 degrees accumulate in the memory, the first image is displayed on the CRT. When the raw data transmitted sequentially at the same angle accumulate, the results of processing for that angle are superimposed on the image and the results of processing of the old data at the same angle are removed simultaneously. By repeating this process, serial CT images are obtained with the minimal delay.

Results: Among patients with grade IV SAH, results were excellent in 8, with mild disability in 14, with severe disability in 1; while the corresponding results for grade V patients who could be treated (n = 19) were: excellent in 2, with mild disability in 1 and severe disability in 4. There were 7 and 12 mortalities for grade IV and V patients respectively, in whom a therapeutic intervention was performed. The factors influencing results included severity of grade of SAH, a poor GCS and JCS score, severity of cisternal hematoma, presence of cerebral edema and herniation. The patients who showed clinical improvement with HBO therapy showed significantly improved outcome following surgical evacuation of the hematoma. However, patients who did not show any clinical improvement with HBO therapy demonstrated poor outcome even when surgery was performed. Conclusions: In patients with poor grade SAH, the advances in therapeutic intervention that have a bearing on the prognosis are studied. In patients with HICH, the usefulness of HBO therapy in selecting patients for surgery and their long term prognostication is discussed. The advantages and limitations of the use of neuroendoscopic evacuation of hematoma under real time CT fluoroscopy (CTF) are also noted.

CT fluoroscopy was possible to evacuate and flush out cerebral hematoma in deep basal ganglia extremely safely and precisely by free hand under CTF guidance and also place an indwelling drainage tube. CTF enabled serial assessment of the status of hematoma removal by evacuation and checking for re-bleeding; cerebral deformation and changes in target position associated with intaoperative CSF leakage and hematoma removal were also detected by CTF. Extremely useful neuro-navigation systems can be constructed by overlaying CT-fluoroscopy as a a real-time monitor on a navigator using digital images and the planning system and by optimizing their combined use.

References

1. Katada K, Anno H, Koga S *et al* (1993) Initial trial with CT fluoroscopy Radiology 190: 662
2. Katada K, Anno H, Ogura Y *et al* (1995) Development and early trials of real-time CT fluoroscopy. Neuroradiology 37: 587–588

Neuropsychological Evaluation of the Patients with Unruptured Cerebral Aneurysms Combined with Asymptomatic Cerebral Infarction Before and after Surgery

A. Fukunaga[1], K. Uchida[1], H. Kashima[2], J. Hashimoto[3], and T. Kawase[1]

[1] Department of Neurosurgery, Keio University, School of Medicine, Tokyo, Japan
[2] Department of Psychiatry, Keio University, School of Medicine, Tokyo, Japan
[3] Department of Radiology, Keio University, School of Medicine, Tokyo, Japan

Objectives: As we have previously reported, neuropsychological function and cerebral blood flow (CBF) often decrease after surgery for unruptured aneurysms of the anterior communicating artery (ACoA) or after surgery for any unruptured cerebral aneurysms (UCA) in patients older than 65 years old but usually recovers to preoperative levels by 3 months after surgery. These findings indicate that operations for UCA are satisfactorily safe and effective, and that such studies can help determine when patients can resume activities of daily life [1]. In addition, we sometimes have opportunities to operate on asymptomatic patients with UCA combined with or without lacuna infarction. Thus, it is very important to investigate how craniotomy affects the higher brain function of these patients.

Methods: Sixteen patients with UCA combined with asymptomatic cerebral infarction (group I) were evaluated comparing to 42 patients with UCA without cerebral infarction (group C). All the patients had no evident neurological deficits before surgery and were operated by pterional approach. Six neuropsychological examinations (Mini-Mental State test, "Kana-hiroi" test, Maze test, Word fluency test, Digit span and Auditory verbal learning tests of 7 words) and SPECT were performed before and after surgery.

Results: Though no patients had neurological deficits after surgery, there was a statistically significant difference between group I (62.5%) and group C (19.3%) in the deteriorating rates in Mini-Mental State test 1 month after surgery (p < 0.05). The 42.9% of group I and the 93.8% of group C recovered at the preoperative neuropsychological level 3 months after surgery, respectively (p < 0.05). In SPECT study, CBF temporarily decreased after surgery, but there was not a significant difference between group I and group C.

Discussion: Retracting the brain with spatulas can reduce local CBF and injure brain parenchyma [2, 3]. The longer brain is retracted during surgery, the more brain parenchyma may be damaged especially in the patients with asymptomatic cerebral infarction, who

may have chronic cerebral ischemia. The CBF is controlled by an autoregulatory system in emergency situations in healthy persons. However, in persons with severe hypotension or arteriosclerosis, the CBF may fail to be maintained because of a failure of autoregulation, resulting in postoperative higher cortical complications.

Conclusions: Patients in group I should be cared to avoid excessive brain retraction or hypotension during surgery and have to be followed up for their higher brain function after surgery, until it recovered completely.

References

1. Fukunaga A *et al* (1999) Neuropsychological evaluation and cerebral blood flow study of 30 patients with unruptured cerebral aneurysms before and after surgery. Surg Neurol 51(2): 132–139
2. Horimoto C *et al* (1990) [Surgical treatment of aged patients with ruptured cerebral aneurysm; evaluation of the operations performed without using retractors.] No shinkei Geka 20: 553–557 (Jpn)
3. Yokoh A *et al* (1983) Intermittent versus continuous brain retraction – an experimental study. J Neurosurg 58: 918–923

Neurological Outcome after Decompressive Craniectomy (DC) in 39 Patients Suffering from Middle Cerebral Artery (MCA) Infarction

T. von Wild, G. H. Schneider, T. Bardt, W. Lanksch, and A. Unterberg

Department Neurosurgery, Charité, Campus Virchow, Humboldt University, Berlin, Germany

Objectives: Cerebral lobe infarction caused by traumatic brain contusion, arterial vascular spasm or occlusion, with malignant brain edema may lead to intracranial hypertension resistant to all medical treatments. In selected cases, DC therefore may be indicated, but is controversial.

Patients and Methods: Our retrospective study included, from 1995 to 1999, 39 patients (19 f, 20 m; age: 56.2 ± 1.7 yrs (23–74) with massive by decompressive hemicraniectomy during the acute stage (6 hrs to 3 day). 14 patients (36%) showed preoperative asymmetry of the pupils. Intracranial pressure (ICP) was monitored in 16 cases. 6 months after decompression, Glasgow Outcome Score (GOS) and functional extended Barthel-Index were assessed.

Results and Conclusion: In 26 (67%) DC effectively reduced intracranial pressure. 6 patients showed cerebral transtentorial herniation despite decompression. 1/3 of the total died.

7 deaths were related to non-neurological causes. 12 patients who died were older than 50 yrs. Only two patients (50 and 55 yrs) could be reintegrated with minimal deficits (GOS 5).

24 patients (61%) were left severely disabled (GOS 3). The mean extended Barthel-Index of survivors was 34.5 ± 22.4 (max. Score: 64). No patient with an infarction volume < 300 cm3 died, though there is no significant correlation between infarct volume and GOS. The functional extended Barthel-Index seems not be influenced by the area of decompression.

References

1. Rieke D (1997) Decompressive surgery in space-occupying hemispheric infarction: result of an open, prospective trial. Care Med 23: 1576–1578
2. Prosiegel M *et al* (1996) Erweiterte Barthel Index. Neurol Rehab 1: 7–13

Sequelae of Damage to Extra-Intracranial Arteries Following Head Injury

F. A. Serbinenko, A. G. Lysachev, L. B. Likhterman, A. A. Potapov, and A. D. Kravtchouk

The Burdenko Neurosurgery Institute, Moscow, Russia

Introduction: Vascular sequelae of head injury have been studied less than tissue and liquorodynamic sequelae [1].

Material and Method: 1042 patients with vascular impairments resulting from head injury were admitted to the Burdenko Neurosurgery Institute from 1970 to 1999. Carotid-cavernous fistulas (89,2%) and pseudoaneurysms (9,2%) were prevalent. In addition to clinical and CT examinations, serial angiography by Seldinger's method was performed before and after surgery.

Results: Clinical manifestation of head and neck vascular impairments' sequelae usually appears after a delay after head injury.

Traumatic Carotid-Cavernous Fistulas: 86,5% of patients underwent internal carotid artery reconstruction using Serbinenko's baloon [2]. 13,5% underwent deconstructive surgery. Mortality rate was 0,3%, disability rate 0,9%. Among 504 patients suffering visual function disorders full recovery was observed in 36,9%, improvement in 20,0%, deterioration in 1,5%, absence of change after surgery in 41,6%. Among 796 patients suffering eye movement disorders, significant improvement was observed in 17,5%, partial improvement in 60,8%, deterioration in 3,3%.

Traumatic Pseudoaneurysms with Massive Epistaxis: endovascular interventions with occlusion of the damaged arteries was performed in 96 patients. Mortality rate was 2,4%, disability rate 10,6%.

Traumatic Arterio-Venous Fistulas of Vertebral Artery: vertebral artery and fistula occlusion with baloon-catheter was performed in 10 patients, vertebral artery reconstruction in 2. All 12 patients recovered.

Conclusion: Endovascular treatment represents an efficient treatment for sequelae of head and neck vascular damage. Reconstructive surgery on be performed in most cases.

References

1. Likhterman LB, Potapov AA, Kravtchouk AD (1999) Clinical classification and conceptual approaches to treatment of head injury sequelae. Voprosy Neurochirurgii 3: 5–10
2. Serbinenko FA (1974) Balloon catheterization and occlusion of major cerebral vessels. J Neurosurg 44: 125–145

Dorsal Column Stimulation for Arousal of Coma

T. Kanno

Department of Neurosurgery, Fujita Health University

Some neurosurgical patients may survive in prolonged coma, even after aggressive treatments such as surgery, ICP control, etc. in the acute stage.

The patients move on to the subacute stage while we, neurosurgeons, generally do not apply any special treatment. For the arousal of coma in the subacute and chronic stage, several new approaches have been developed in the last 10 years, i.e. dorsal column stimulations, deep brain stimulation, median nerve stimulation and vagal nerve stimulation. The action mechanism of these treatments for arousal of coma has already been verified neurophysiologically and neurochemically. Stimulation is given to reticular formation and

thalamic nuclei, which enhances the secretion of chemical substances such as catecholamine, GABA, prostaglandin, acetylcholine, etc. Then it causes the enhancement of cortical function.

The authors have experienced the dorsal column stimulation in 131 patients during last decade. Clinical improvement was obtained in 42% of the cases. A summary of the results will be given below.

Cases: In a total of 131 cases the persistent vegetative state was treated by dorsal column stimulation (DCS) during 1985 to 1999. Mean periods of vegetative state were 11.1 months. None of them did show an improvement before starting DCS. Ninety of the patients were male, 41 were female. Causes for vegetative state were trauma in 65 cases, anoxia in 28, cerebrovascular disease in 25 and others (brain tumor, etc.) in 13.

Procedure: Bilateral stimulation of dorsal column with epidural electrodes inserted between C2 and C3.

Stimuli were constant voltage pulses at 3.0 volts, duration 0.2 milliseconds, 50 Hz, amp 7, delivered continuously between 8am–8pm.

Observations: Effective response was observed in 56 patients. Among the 56 cases, 18 showed response to verbal order, speak, and oral intake of foods. More effective results were observed in patients of age under 35 (62.5%) and in trauma cases (91.1%).

Studies of SPECT, CT, EEG, and catecholamine metabolism in CSF were performed. Effective cases showed an increase in $\hat{I}^3CBF$ and CMRO2 during ongoing DCS. It is not known whether these changes outlasted the stimulation period.

EEG changes: Alpha activation and delta decrease persisted for 60 minutes post-DCS.

Neurochemistry: DCS increased catecholamine metabolism. Acetylcholine increased in CSF, FDG metabolism and $\hat{I}^3CBF$ increases were found with PET and SPECT in 42% of the patients but no effect in the remaining 58%. Comparisons between the improved and not-improved groups indicated that cases involving those lacking large low-density defects on head CT, those without severe damage to the thalamus, and those without marked cerebral atrophy in which the $\hat{I}^3CBF$ is more than 20 ml/min/100 gm, are good candidates for DCS. It is speculated that in cases with some potential for neurologic improvement (young age, less abnormal findings on CT), DCS enhances catecholamine metabolism and increases $\hat{I}^3CBF$ leading to better EEG and clinical improvement.

Hence the following indication for selection: young age, TBI, no marked atrophy, no thalamic involvement, preserved thalamocortical fibers, $\hat{I}^3CBF$ greater than 20 cc/min.

Patients with Prolonged Consciousness Disturbances and Brain Electrical Stimulation Therapy

J. Ciurea[1], A. V. Ciurea[1], Ileana Simoca[1], R. Perin[1], D. Mircea[1], and Al. Constantinovici[1]

[1] Neurosurgical Department, "Prof. Dr. D. Bagdasar" Clinical Emergency Hospital
[2] Neurology Department, "Prof. Dr. D. Bagdasar" Clinical Emergency Hospital

Introduction: Vegetative state (VS) diagnosis is time dependent ("after three months ...") and involve major medical and social resources. Neurorehabilitation has a paramount position in this management.

From a total of 24, brain electrical stimulation therapy (BEST) was performed in 14 patients; ten were excluded due to different complications starting simultaneously with stimulation (pulmonary, urine infection and skin trophic lesions). All the other 14 presented prolonged consciousness disturbances and were introduced in a complex protocol including conventional drug therapies, physiotherapy, etc. One electrode was placed in cavum and the other on vertex. The frequency was variable (4–200 Hz) and the voltage from 1 to 10 V. A traumatic history was found in 12 patients, a vascular in one and a tumoral in one patient. Age ranged between 17 to 70 years. There were 6 female and 8 male patients. Glasgow Coma Scale, Glasgow Outcome Score and Ohata scale were used for assessment. CT scan was used for brain injury assessment and EEG for follow-up. Time elapsed from admittance to start of stimulation was about 30 days. Time of stimulation varied from 5 hours to 40 days. The non-traumatic cases were not followed-up due to objective causes.

Results: A favourable outcome was recorded in 9 traumatic patients of twelve. A restless and confusion period was recorded in two patients. Three deaths were due as follows: two to pulmonary complications and one to an apalic syndrome.

Discussions: Brain stimulation has been used successfully before as it is presented in the literature. The action mechanisms are still at hypothetical level. This study focuses on "preventive" approach of potential candidates to VS. BEST correlated with an on line EEG spectral analysis will open new perspectives in neuromodulation understanding and use as a "more physiological" therapeutical device.

Conclusion: the used method seems to be a useful tool in available armamentarium for treatment of prolonged consciousness disturbances.

Vigilance Enhancing Effect of Botulinum Toxin A (Btx A) after Local Application in Vegetative Patients with Severe Spasticity Following Traumatic Brain Injury (TBI)

Th. Paehge, Th. Sprenkel, and K. von Wild

Neurosurgical Clinic, Clemenshospital, Münster, Germany

Objectives: Prolonged coma, unawareness and spasticity are the main problems in Neurorehabilitation of patients after severe TBI. Early local application of Btx A may be indicated when physical therapy could not prevent contractures due to painful central spasticity. Central effects of Btx A on higher brain functions are not reported so far.

Method: Botulinum Toxin A (Botox®, Dysport®) is locally applied according to the literature in patients after severe TBI, however the exact timing for the initial treatment is still being discussed. We perform an interdisciplinary approach together with our physio- and vocational therapists and nurses in our department on posttraumatic neurorehabilitation.

Results: Surprisingly we observed a central effect with an improvement in consciousness, attention and awareness after the first and only single local application of Btx A in two of our vegetative patients in between ten days which lasted permanently. This was assessed with the aid of the Coma Remission Scale with an increase of the score up to the maximum of 24 points.

Discussion: Central effects of Btx A on higher nervous functions, concomitant to the reduction of the central muscle spasticity, have not been reported so far except for one personal report by Ortega-Suhrkamp (1999). This effect after some days may be due to a reduction of pain and at the same time suppression of the activating system of the formatio reticularis mesencephali. One may speculate in addition upon a release of acethylcholine secondary to an improvement of CBF of the brain stem, as this was demonstrated earlier by our group for pyritinol (Encephabol®). These findings have to be evaluated prospectively.

Reference

1. Wissel, J *et al* (2000) Management of spasticity associated pain with Botulinum toxin A. J Pain Symptom Management: 20(1): 44–49

Post-Traumatic Epilepsy and Two-Year MRI Follow-up of Head Trauma: A Prospective Study

G. Polonara[1], M. Signorino[2], A. Messori[1], F. Angeleri[2], and U. Salvolini[1]

[1] Department of Neuroradiology, University of Ancona, Ancona, Italy

[2] Department of Neurology, University of Ancona, Ancona, Italy

Introduction: Post-traumatic epilepsy (PTE) affects the outcome of head injury (HI). We correlate the evolution of cerebral lesions with Magnetic Resonance Imaging (MRI) with the PTE onset.

Goals: To identify the best sequences to follow the evolution of traumatic brain lesions, and to investigate how the presence of haemosiderin and gliosis and the onset of PTE are correlated.

Methods: 185 consecutively enrolled HI adult in-patients were evaluated in the acute phase after trauma by using clinical examination, EEG, CT, and MRI when possible. The examination protocol, with MRI instead of CT, was repeated within 6–8 weeks, 12–14 weeks, 1 year, and 2 years, respectively. 113 patients have completed the examination protocol.

Results: GE T2* was found more sensitive than TSE in haemosiderin detection. Gliosis was better demonstrated with turbo-FLAIR in most cases, and turbo-FLAIR was never found inferior to TSE in detecting it. Multiple shearing injuries were well detectable as haemosiderin spots with GE T2* 1 month after trauma; their visibility increased during the first 3–4 months, and they became less conspicuous during the 1st or 2nd year.

The evolution of brain contusions towards gliosis and/or porencephaly usually began at the 6th week and was more conspicuous at 2–3 months. After 1 year the lesion appeared smaller and better delimited and the adjacent subarachnoid spaces were clearly dilated. Haemosiderin deposits within the gliotic-porencephalic lesion were detected in some cases by both GE T2* and TSE up to the 4th month, only by GE T2* thereafter.

11 of the 109 patients developed PTE. Focal gliosis with or without haemosiderin as shown by MRI one year after trauma was significantly correlated with PTE.

Conclusion: GE T2* and turbo-FLAIR sequences are recommended in the late follow-up studies of HI patients. Focal gliosis is a risk factor for PTE, whether it includes haemosiderin spots or not. Haemosiderin spots without gliosis do not seem to play a role in developing PTE.

Characteristics of Emotional Personality Disturbances in Adolescents with Chronic Post-Traumatic Headaches (CPTH) after Mild Traumatic Brain Injury (MTBI)

V. V. Belopassov and I. G. Ismaiiova

Department of Neurology, Astrakhan State Medical Academy, Bakinskaya, Astrakhan, Russia

Emotional-personally disturbances in 71 adolescents with CPTH after MTBI have been studied. Methods of investigation: pathocharacterologic inquiry by A. Ye. Lichko, test of Spielberger, Beck. Control group: 24 adolescents after MTBI without CPTH.

In adolescents with CPTH accentuation of character, more often of epileptoid, hysteroid, unstable, psychoasthenic and mixed types has been discovered. Low conformity, delinquency, risk of social dysfunction, psychopathy were not uncommon. Adolescents with CPTH were characterized by high sensitivity, affective explosiveness, emotional – will liability, the state of malicious – dreary mood, depressive and demonstrative features, distorted self-evaluation, sense of inferiority, asthenic type of psychologic defence, tendency to be hypochondriacal, self-analysis, instability interests, low ego-strength, insufficient initiative, indecision, anxious mistrustfulness, egocentrism, falsity.

In adolescents without CPTH accentuations of character are discovered only in half cases, mainly of the hyperthymic type. Harmonised development of an individual, balanced emotional background, high ego-strength, low level of anxiety, adequate self-evaluation, proper understanding of the current situation and perspectives, sufficient social activity and maturity, corresponding to age, communicability, sufficient degree af social adaptation. Absence of hypochondric and depressive features, infantile tendencies, heteroaggression, demonstrativeness and falsity are very peculiar to them.

The acquired data prove the essential role of emotional-personality disturbances in the development of CPTH. Hypochondric, demonstrative, depressive, dependent, aggressive personalities are associated with a chronic course of pain syndrome after MTBI. Early identification and psychotherapeutic correction of emotional-personality disturbances in MTBI adolescents, make it possible to optimize rehabilitation, to better social adaptation and life quality. Use of Tanakan decreases the evidence of subjective, asthenia-vegetative, cognitive and ernotional disturbances after MTBI.

References

1. Mudrova O (1995) A Vegetative regulations in different periods of cranial traumas in children: clinical and psychophysiological analysis. Ivanovo Thesis
2. Abramov VA (1986) J Neurol Psychiatry 86: 562–567

Longterm Neuropsychological Outcome after Childhood Traumatic Brain Injury (TBI): Effects of Age at Injury

B. Benz, A. Ritz, and S. Kiesow
NRZ Friedehorst, Bremen, Germany

Introduction: Cerebral plasticity has long been believed to have beneficial effects in cases of pediatric TBI, in contrast to observations of delayed onset of symptoms, known as "growing into a deficit".

Method: In a long-term follow-up study, former patients of a neurological rehabilitation centre are reassessed at least 3 years after trauma. In the present sample (n = 106), mean age at follow-up is 19 years, 9 years after trauma. Subjects had suffered TBI between 2,5 and 15,11 years, with a mean age at injury of 9 years and severe trauma in 61% of cases. Effects of severity and age at injury on relevant neuropsychological functions were analysed.

Results: Trauma severity alone affected speed of information processing ($p < .0001$) and visuo-spatial performance ($p < .007$). Additional age-at-trauma effects emerged for attentional functions ($p < .04$), memory ($p < .005$) and verbal competence ($p < .0002$).

Executive skills were only related to age at trauma ($p < .012$). Patients with scores < 1 SD below the reference mean in this domain were more severely impaired on neuropsychological measures, with both lower and more discrepant IQ scores (WISC-RV-IQ/P-IQ: 73/62 vs. 94/91).

Conclusion: Age at trauma is an important variable acting upon both quantitative and qualitative aspects of outcome, pointing to an increased risk for those who suffer disruption of cerebral development early in life.

References

1. Anderson V, Moore C (1995) Age at injury as a predictor of outcome following pediatric head injury: a longitudinal perspective. Child Neuropsychol 1/3: 187–202
2. Benz B, Ritz A, Kiesow S (1999) Influence of age-related factors on long-term outcome after traumatic brain injury (TBI) in children: a review of recent literature and some preleminary findings. Restorative Neurol Neurosci 14(2/3): 135–143
3. Taylor G, Alden J (1997) Age-related differences in outcomes following childhood brain insults: an introduction and overview. J Int Neuropsychol Soc (JINS) 3: 555–567

Suicide Following Traumatic Brain Injury: A Population Study

T. W. Teasdale[1], A. A. W. Engberg[2], and T. W. Teasdale[3]
[1] Department of Psychology, University of Copenhagen, Denmark
[2] Division of Stroke, Hidovre University Hospital, University of Copenhagen, Copenhagen, Denmark
[3] Department of Psychology, University of Copenhagen, Copenhagen, Denmark

Introduction: Although the potential risk of suicide following a traumatic brain injury is clinically recognised, most reports in the literature have concerned only small numbers of cases.

Goals: To establish the incidence of suicide among a large population-derived cohort of brain-injured patients over a follow-up time-period of up to 15 years.

Methods: From a Danish population register of hospitalisations covering the years 1979–1993, patients were selected who had suffered either a concussion (n = 110 289), a cranial fracture (n = 6 573) or a cerebral contusion and/or traumatic intracranial haemorrhage (n = 8 529). Concussion patients were included as a control group for the more severe injunes. Deaths were identified in a national register of causes of death.

Results: In the three diagnostic groups, there had been respectively 717 (0.65%), 44 (0.67%) and 87 (0.83%) cases of suicide. Comparing the three groups, Cox regression analyses for proportional hazards indicated there is a relatively elevated risk for suicide following a cerebral contusion/traumatic intracranial haemorrhage among males (hazard ratio = 1.4 relative to the concussion group) but not among females. For such males, the suicide risk is related to the length of hospitalisation, but not to time since injury.

Conclusion: The often drastic psychological and social consequences of a severe TBI can lead a male patient to suicide. The increased risk is small. That this effect is not present for women is probably related to the lower rate of suicides among them.

Attentional Complaints of Professionals are More Accurate than Patients' and Relatives' Complaints Following Severe Traumatic Brain Injury

M. Leclercq, G. Deloche, and M. Rousseaux

Service de Rééducation Neurologique – Hopital Swynghedauw, Lille, France

Introduction: The aim of this study was to perform a direct comparison of the patients', close relatives', and professionals' perception of attention disorders following cerebral injury (traumatic: TBI; or cerebrovascular: CVA), and to confront these perceptions with the effective performance.

Patients and Methods: 91 patients with TBI (49) or CVA (42) were recruited. Both groups were similar. A modified version of the Ponsford and kinsella attention questionnaire (16 + 1 questions) was presented to the patients (auto-evaluation), close relatives and close therapists (hetero-evaluations), and to 91 normal control subjects. Objective attention disorders were assessed with the TAP Battery (Zimmermann).

Results: Subjective attention disorders were more severe in CVA than in TBI patients and controls, in that order (ANOVA; $p < .05$). However, for the hetero-evaluation, complaints were more important following TBI, and the difference with the auto-evaluation was more severe for the therapists' evaluations. Correlations between the auto-evaluation and the instrumental assessments of attention disorders were not significant in TBI patients, when they were frequently so in CVA patients. Furthermore, correlations between the hetero-evaluations from therapists and attention performances were much more significant.

Discussion: Attention disorders were underestimated by TBI but not by CVA patients, due to impaired awareness. The hetero-evaluation is better correlated with objective findings.

Divided Attention after Severe Diffuse Traumatic Brain Injury

J. Couillet, M. Leclercq, M. Rousseaux, Y. Martin, and P. Azouvi

Service de Rééducation Neurologique, Hôpital Raymond Poincaré, Garches, France

Background: Survivors of a severe traumatic brain injury (TBI) often complain of a difficulty in doing two things simultaneously. However, experimental data on divided attention have given conflicting results [1, 2].

Subjects and Methods: 42 severe TBI patients at the subacute or chronic stage performed two tasks under single- and dual-tasks conditions: a) random generation; b) a go-no go task. Moreover, two additional dual-task conditions were given, in which subjects were alternatively asked to focus preferentially on each one of the two simultaneous tasks. Patients were compared to matched controls.

Results: A disproportionate increase of reaction time in the go-no go task under dual-task condition was found in the TBI group, as compared to controls. However, patients were able to modify, at least in part, their pattern of performance in dual-task conditions, according to the specific instructions concerning the task to emphasize.

Discussion: These results confirm previous findings [2, 3] on a divided attention deficit of severe TBI patients. However, they also suggest that patients have a relatively preserved ability to allocate their attentional resources according to task requirements. These

data will be discussed within the van Zomeren and Brouwer (1) model of attention.

References

1. Van Zomeren AH, Brouwer WH (1994) Clinical neuropsychology of attention. Oxford University Press, New York
2. Azouvi P, Jokic C, Van der Linden M, Marlier N, Bussel B (1996) Working memory and supervisory control after severe closed head injury. A study of dual task performance and random generation. J Clin Exp Neuropsychol 18: 317–337
3. Leclercq M, Couillet J, Azouvi P *et al* (in press) Dual task performance after severe traumatic brain injury or vascular prefrontal damage. J Clin Exp Neuropsychol

An Ecological Approach of a Dysexecutive Syndrome

M. Chevignard[1], P. Pradat-Diehl[2], B. Pillon[3], C. Taillefer[1], S. Rousseau[1], C. Le Bras[2], and B. Dubois[3]

[1] Service de Rééducation Neurologique, Hôpital de Ia Salpêtrière, Paris, France

[2] INSERM U289, Hôpital de Ia Salpêtrière, Paris, France

[3] Service de Neurologie, Hôpital de Ia Salpêtrière, Paris, France

Objective: planning is disturbed in patients with frontal lobe lesions. It refers to the ability to predetermine a course of actions and to monitor its execution according to environmental contingencies.

Therefore, planning difficulties would be better evaluated by script execution of daily life activities than by laboratory tests. The objectives were to test the validity of script execution as a predictor of planning difficulties in daily life.

Design/Methods: script execution and generation were compared in 11 patients with a dysexecutive syndrome due CT or MRI defined frontal lesions. Age: 35.4 (SD 12.3) years; education: 13.8 (3.4) years and 10 matched controls, using 3 scripts: (1) shopping for groceries; (2) cooking: (3) answering a letter and finding the way to mail it. For each script, 2 examiners followed the patient and quoted behavior. The dysexecutive syndrome was also investigated with cognitive tests (Wisconsin CST; Tower of London Task; Six Elements Tests; Trail Making Test; verbal fluency; verbal learning) and behavioral scales.

Results: two way ANOVAs showed ($p < 0.01$) more errors in script execution than generation and in patients than in controls; the difference execution/generation was greater in patients. Furthermore, «lack of context analysis» and «environmental adherence» best differentiated patients from controls. Finally the number of errors in execution correlated with the score on behavioral questionnaires.

Conclusion: these results suggest that script execution is a valid approach to estimate the severity of planning deficits in daily life activities.

References

1. Chevignard M, Pradat-Diehl P, Pillon B, Taillefer C, Rousseau S, Le Bras C, Dubois B. An ecological approach of a dysexecutive syndrome, Cortex (in press)
2. Sirigu A, Zalla T, Grafman J, Agid Y, Dubois B (1995) Selective impairments in managerial knowledge following prefrontal cortex damage. Cortex 31: 301–316

Quality of Life 2 to 6 Years after Severe Traumatic Brain Injury (TBI)

L. Mailhan, P. Azouvi, J. L. Truelle, and A. Dazord
Department of Neurological Rehabilitation, Raymond Poincaré Hospital, Garches, France

Objective: To assess satisfaction with life of severe TBI patients and their families.

Patients and Methods: 50 patients hospitalised in a rehabilitation department after severe TBI from 1993 to 1995 were included. Quality of life was assessed by the Subjective Quality of Life Profile (SQLP) [1].

Patients rated their satisfaction on a 5-point scale for 39 items related to various domains (e.g. interpersonal relationships, leisure and vocational activities...). These data were compared to ratings made by a close relative. Quality of life data were compared to impairments, disability and handicap.

Results: Patients' satisfaction was globally low, particularly for items related to cognitive functions, physical abilities and self-esteem. Families' ratings of patients' satisfaction were parallel but lower than patients' ratings. Patients' satisfaction was significantly correlated with motor impairments, anxiety level, basic and advanced ADL, vocational status, and the Glasgow Outcome Scale.

Discussion and Conclusion: Severe TBI patients two to six years post injury demonstrated a relatively poor satisfaction with life. Satisfaction appeared to be affected by the presence of motor rather than cognitive impairments, and was significantly related to functional and vocational status.

References

1. Dazord A, Gerin P, Boissel J (1994) Subjective quality of life assessment in therapeutic trials: Presentation of a new instrument in France (SQLP: Subjective quality of life profile) and first results. In: Orley J, Kuyken W (eds) Quality of life assessments: international perspectives. Springer, Berlin Heidelberg New York Tokyo, p 185–195

Author Index

Index of Keywords

SpringerMedicine

R. W. Seiler,

H.-J. Steiger (eds.)

Cerebral Vasospasm

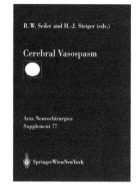

2001. XI, 269 pages. 90 figures, partly in colour.

Hardcover **EUR 108,–**

Reduced price for subscribers

to "Acta Neurochirurgica": **EUR 97,20**

(Recommended retail prices)

All prices are net-prices subject to local VAT.

ISBN 3-211-83650-0

Acta Neurochirurgica, Supplementum 77

Cerebral vasospasm remains a major clinical problem in patients with sub-arachnoid hemorrhage. Neuroprotection with calcium antagonists, hemo-dynamic therapy and interventional angioplasty have an established role in the management of this disease, but an effective single drug for prevention or treatment of the vasospasm is still lacking.

This book contains selected contributions to the 7th International Conference on Cerebral Vasospasm held in Interlaken, Switzerland, in June 2000. Part I of the book concentrates on basic science and experimental vasospasm. The molecular biology of vasospasm, the role of endothelin and nitric oxide as well as the potential of gene therapy are presented.

Part II concentrates on the diagnosis and therapy of clinical vasospasm. New diagnostic tools are presented, including diffusion and perfusion-weighted MRI, MR spectroscopy and microdialysis with metabolic monitoring. Leaders in the field discuss the current indications and results of endovascular treatment of cerebral vasospasm. The latter chapters are devoted to the treatment of clinical vasospasm with new drugs and to the prevention and treatment of ischemic deficits with neuroprotective drugs and hemodynamic therapy. The book provides the state of the art in the major subjects of the molecular biology of vasoconstriction and experimental vasospasm as well as the diagnosis and treatment of clinical vasospasm.

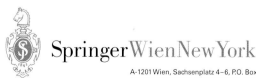

Springer WienNew York

A-1201 Wien, Sachsenplatz 4–6, P.O. Box 89, Fax +43.1.330 24 26, e-mail: books@springer.at, Internet: **www.springer.at**
D-69126 Heidelberg, Haberstraße 7, Fax +49.6221.345-229, e-mail: orders@springer.de
USA, Secaucus, NJ 07096-2485, P.O. Box 2485, Fax +1.201.348-4505, e-mail: orders@springer-ny.com
Eastern Book Service, Japan, Tokyo 113, 3–13, Hongo 3-chome, Bunkyo-ku, Fax +81.3.38 18 08 64, e-mail: orders@svt-ebs.co.jp

SpringerMedicine

Hans-Jakob Steiger,

Eberhard Uhl (eds.)

Risk Control and Quality Management in Neurosurgery

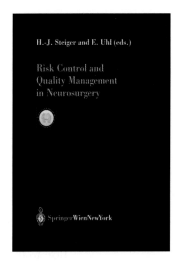

2001. IX, 227 pages. 45 figures.
Hardcover EUR 108,–
ISBN 3-211-83678-0
Acta Neurochirurgica, Supplementum 78

Quality in an invasive discipline such as neurosurgery comprises evidence based medicine, cost effectiveness and also risk control. Risk control and quality management have become a science on their own, combining the expertise of many specialists such as psychologists, mathematicians and also economists. Intensive communication with basic safety scientists as well as safety experts from the industry and traffic promises ideas and concepts than can be adopted for neurosurgery.

An international conference was held in Munich in October 2000 bringing together neurosurgeons and safety experts from outside medicine in order to discuss basic aspects of risk control and quality management and to develop structures applicable to neurosurgery. Basic aspects such as principles of risk and safety management, the human factor as well as standards of neurosurgical patient care, proficiency of staff and residents, and industrial quality standards were discussed. The presentations and discussions resulted in a wealth of new ideas and concepts. This book contains this material and thus provides a unique and comprehensive source of information on the current possibilities of quality management in neurosurgery.

Contents:

Preface. • Basics. • The Human Factor. • Principles of Quality Management in Medicine. • Standards of Perioperative Care. • Learning from Errors in Neurosurgery. • Proficiency of Staff and Residents. • Risk and Quality Management in research. • ISO 9000 Quality Concepts Applied to Neurosurgery. • Risk Control and Quality Management in the next century

(Recommended retail prices)

All prices are net-prices subject to local VAT.

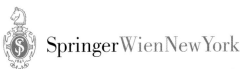
Springer WienNewYork

A-1201 Wien, Sachsenplatz 4–6, P.O. Box 89, Fax +43.1.330 24 26, e-mail: books@springer.at, Internet: **www.springer.at**
D-69126 Heidelberg, Haberstraße 7, Fax +49.6221.345-229, e-mail: orders@springer.de
USA, Secaucus, NJ 07096-2485, P.O. Box 2485, Fax +1.201.348-4505, e-mail: orders@springer-ny.com
Eastern Book Service, Japan, Tokyo 113, 3–13, Hongo 3-chome, Bunkyo-ku, Fax +81.3.38 18 08 64, e-mail: orders@svt-ebs.co.jp

Springer-Verlag
and the Environment

WE AT SPRINGER-VERLAG FIRMLY BELIEVE THAT AN international science publisher has a special obligation to the environment, and our corporate policies consistently reflect this conviction.

WE ALSO EXPECT OUR BUSINESS PARTNERS – PRINTERS, paper mills, packaging manufacturers, etc. – to commit themselves to using environmentally friendly materials and production processes.

THE PAPER IN THIS BOOK IS MADE FROM NO-CHLORINE pulp and is acid free, in conformance with international standards for paper permanency.